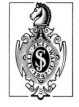

Henry T. Lynch   Petre Tautu (Eds.)

Recent Progress in the
Genetic Epidemiology
of Cancer

With 19 Figures

Springer-Verlag
Berlin Heidelberg New York
London Paris Tokyo
Hong Kong Barcelona

HENRY T. LYNCH, MD, Professor of Medicine
Professor and Chairman
Department of Preventive Medicine/Public Health
Creighton University Medical School
California & 24th Street
Omaha, Nebraska 68178, USA

PETRE TAUTU, MD, Professor
Institut für Epidemiologie und Biometrie
Deutsches Krebsforschungszentrum
Im Neuenheimer Feld 280
W-6900 Heidelberg, FRG

ISBN 3-540-53022-3 Springer-Verlag Berlin Heidelberg New York
ISBN 0-387-53022-3 Springer-Verlag New York Berlin Heidelberg

Library of Congress Cataloging-in-Publication Data. Recent progress in the genetic epidemiology of cancer / H.T. Lynch, P. Tautu (eds.). p. cm. Includes bibliographical references and index. ISBN 3-540-53022-3 (alk. paper). − ISBN 0-387-53022-3 (alk. paper) 1. Cancer − Genetic aspects. 2. Cancer − Epidemiology. 3. Genetic epidemiology. I. Lynch, Henry T. II. Tautu, Petre. [DNLM: 1. Neoplasms − epidemiology. 2. Neoplasms − genetics. QZ 202 R294] RC268.4.R43 1991 616.99′4042-dc20 DNLM/DLC for Library of Congress 90-10378 CIP

© Springer-Verlag Berlin Heidelberg 1991
Printed in Germany

Typesetting: International Typesetters Inc., Makati, Philippines
21/3130-543210 − Printed on acid-free paper

Preface

The discipline of genetic epidemiology pertains to the vertical transmission of the susceptibility (predisposition) to a complex disease in a structured population. This statement meets halfway the broad definition given by N.E. Morton and S.C. Chung in 1978[1] and the concise one given by M.-C. King et al. in 1984[2]. It pinpoints the fundamental genetic hypothesis, namely, the existence of an inherited condition that predisposes an individual to a specific disease, and the corresponding subject of investigation, the family. Thus, the genetic epidemiological situation consists of three basic elements: (1) the genealogical structure, (2) the mode of inheritance (i.e., the "genetic model") for the trait of interest, and (3) the observable phenotypes of susceptibility.

It is clear that genetic epidemiology is a research field positioned at the intersection of molecular genetics, population genetics, and clinical genetics. Perhaps the genealogical tree should be its central element: it evidences something forgotten in molecular genetics, namely the relationships, and associations with probabilistic and statistical concepts from population genetics. It offers a structure and a "history" for those clinicians studying familial diseases who are searching for genetic determinants of susceptibility. The genetic epidemiologist begins his analysis with a point on this genealogical tree, namely the proband, and attempts to carry out (nonrandom) "ascertainment sampling" by using a strategy that depends on the form and dimension (extended pedigrees versus nuclear families) of the tree. The important quality of a genealogical structure is the information (hopefully of high accuracy) that it provides about nonobservable genotypes underlying the observed phenotypes; a certain criterion of sampling optimality is required which is dependent on the postulated

---

[1] "Genetic epidemiology is concerned with etiology, distribution and control of disease in relatives and with inherited causes of disease in populations" (Morton NE, Chung CS, 1978. Preface. In: Genetic epidemiology. Academic, New York).

[2] "Genetic epidemiology is the study of how and why diseases cluster in families and ethnic groups" (King MC et al. 1984. Genetic epidemiology. Annu Rev Public Health 5:1–32).

inheritance model. It should also be stressed that, from a clinical point of view, the "observed phenotype" is, at least in the first step, vaguely defined: "cancer," with any of its localizations, is only a collective label for many clinical entities.

Many inherited disorders of man display phenotypes for which adequate biochemical explanations or markers are lacking. Often there are no animal models that faithfully mimic the human disease (for example, the hereditary renal carcinoma in the rat is a unique, specific, hereditary cancer). In such situations, one must apply *reverse genetics*, that is, "the isolation of a gene without reference to a specific protein or without any reagents or functional assay useful in its detection"[3], or, in other words, the use of genetic linkage with empirically chosen markers. Obviously, this is only an ingenuous approximation. In the words of F. Hecht (1990), "Once reverse genetics has had its day, forward genetics must again move ahead to learn how each gene acts to produce the final phenotype."[4]

Does there exist such a thing as "reverse epidemiology" which is predicated on the following strategy: find the gene first, and use this to define both the population at risk and the class of environmental agents involved? Ataxia-telangiectasia (AT) may be a good example: physical mapping of the chromosome region 11q23 led to localization of the AT gene. The healthy heterozygous carriers can be detected. However, the external factor(s) require elucidation. The remaining scientific problem is cogent to *forward genetics*: one has to consider either (1) the existence of a path from the AT gene to immunodeficiency and thence to neoplasia, (2) a predisposition in heterozygotes to cancer at certain sites, e.g., the breast in young females, or (3) an indirect way in homozygotes by increasing the risk of malignancy.

This example raises an important distinction. In 1990, T.A. Sellers and coworkers reported evidence for Mendelian inheritance in the pathogenesis of lung cancer, introducing supplementary data on tobacco consumption and employment history as environmental covariates. In fact, the opposition gene–environment is, like many other conceptual oppositions, a rigid one and it is difficult to dissect transmissible environmental and cultural factors from true genetic factors. In practice, "general" epidemiology includes genetic factors among other defined external factors and applies its specific methodology, whereas genetic epidemiology subsumes environmental effects under the concepts of "reduced penetrance" and "sporadics." The

[3]   Orkin SH (1986) Reverse genetics and human disease. Cell 47:845–850.
[4]   Hecht F (1990) Genetic linkage and physical mapping of a cancer gene. Ataxia-telangiectasia (Editorial). Cancer Genet Cytogenet 46:133–134.

remarkable regressive models introduced by G. Bonney and colleagues can detect and estimate major gene effects, but without postulating explicit genetic and environmental causal mechanisms (although these can, however, be incorporated by choosing suitable parameters).

If we refer to human neoplasias, we must note that the temporal sequence of genetic alterations is still unknown, so there are serious difficulties in identifying those putative loci responsible for "primary cancer susceptibility." New reports show that chromosome regions 13q and 11p15 are not the sites of a primary lesion for breast cancer, but R. Kumar and coworkers demonstrate that activation of *ras* oncogenes can precede the onset of neoplasia and that they can exist in apparently normal cells for long periods of time without inducing malignant transformations.

The power of linkage analysis of complex traits is that it provides a collection of statistical techniques useful to prove some genetic hypotheses. Of particular interest may be the recent techniques based on essential concepts of population genetics, such as the concept of "identity" of a gene: two genes can be identical "in state" or "by descent." The latter concept specifies a transmission process but the former can be useful for markers that are not totally informative.

The complexity of the genetic situations and the diversity of models in genetic epidemiology mean that numerical experiments are necessary, not only for comparing techniques but also for simulating the vertical gene transmission process. *In numero* experiments with random walks on the genetic states of a pedigree should be extended to other adequately random processes, including also demographic and social mechanisms. It is hoped that this approach will develop in a systematic manner in full accord with the genetic-epidemiologic modeling process proposed in this book.

The genetic epidemiology of human neoplasias is going through a period of rapid and dynamic progress. The contributions in this volume, based on a symposium held on 22–23 January 1990 in Heidelberg, should provide the reader with a *tour d'horizon* on the main problems in the genetic epidemiology of cancer. We are indebted to the generous sponsors, the German Cancer Research Center, Heidelberg, Knoll AG, Ludwigshafen, and Boehringer Mannheim GmbH, who made possible this excellent meeting.

HENRY T. LYNCH
PETRE TAUTU

Contents

III. Computer Applications

List of Contributors

You will find the address of each first mentioned author at the beginning of the respective contribution.

I. Introduction

Genetics of Common Tumors

H.T. LYNCH and J.F. LYNCH[1]

Introduction

Host factors play an exceedingly important role in virtually all forms of cancer. A significant question is: "Are there *any* cancers, including those which are clearly sporadic by virtue of a negative family history of cancer through two or more generations, that would not be appropriate for discussion about potential genetic etiology?" A comment by J. Michael Bishop (1986) is appropriate for consideration in answering this question:

Much of contemporary cancer research is motivated by the conviction that cancer is at its heart a genetic disease. This conviction has three main origins: the perception of sometimes vague, sometimes dramatic hereditary diatheses to cancer; the presence of chromosomal damage in at least some cancer cells; and the efforts to equate mutagenic potential to carcinogenicity. Now the conviction has acquired the substance of experiment. Vertebrate cells contain a set of genes that can become tumorigenic "oncogenes" when transduced into retroviruses (Bishop 1983). In their normal guise, these "proto-oncogenes" may be part of the genetic wiring that directs the growth and development of normal cells. And it requires only an easy leap of faith to imagine that these same genes might also be important substrates for carcinogenic influences of diverse sorts.

Advances in genetic epidemiology at the infrahuman and human levels since the turn of the century (and particularly during the past decade) mandate that one embrace the concept that cancer etiology is an exceedingly complex, multistep process involving both genetic and environmental factors. The quantitative and qualitative contribution of genetics and environment to cancer causality in any individual patient can only be approximated crudely. Careful consideration must be given to the specific histologic type of tumor, its usual age of onset, the racial, ethnic, sociocultural, and even the geographic background of the patient. Appropriate division must be made between those cancers characteristic of childhood (retinoblastoma, Wilms' tumor, neuroblastoma), those of adolescence and early adulthood, those which show bimodal age peaks such as Hodgkin's lymphoma, those of middle age, and those of more advanced ages, such as carcinoma of the prostate or multiple myeloma.

[1] Department of Preventive Medicine/Public Health, Creighton University School of Medicine, Omaha, NE 68178, USA

H.T. Lynch and P. Tautu (Eds.)
Recent Progress
in the Genetic Epidemiology of Cancer
© Springer-Verlag Berlin Heidelberg 1991

It seems logical that primary genetic factors must play a greater etiologic role in childhood tumors as opposed to those occurring at an advanced age. This is important when considering the shorter time for environmental exposures to the target cell/organ, such as the retinocytes in a patient destined to develop retinoblastoma. This contrasts to cells of the pleura or mesentery which, after only a limited exposure to asbestos and following a long latency period (30–45 years), may transform into malignant mesothelioma. More common examples would include heavy and prolonged cigarette smoking in the case of bronchogenic carcinoma or heavy sunlight exposure (severe burns with blistering) in childhood and youth followed by the emergence of malignant melanoma in adulthood.

It is important to note that only a fraction of individuals who are exposed to environmental carcinogens develop cancer, e.g., only a few heavy cigarette smokers develop bronchogenic carcinoma. An even smaller fraction of patients exposed to asbestos develop mesothelioma. Why is it then that so many patients with heavy carcinogenic exposure remain cancer-free? A plausible explanation is that the genotype may determine the variable predisposition to cancer through differing cellular phenotypes that are resistant in the one extreme, while in the other, show susceptibility to a given carcinogen. Gradations between profound cancer resistance vs susceptibility would likely characterize the bulk of the population. At the infrahuman level, this logic has been appreciated by geneticists (Heston 1974) since the turn of the century. More recently, in humans, an extraordinary interhuman variation in susceptibility to carcinogens has been investigated, consonant with the concept of ecogenetics (Mulvihill 1984). Indeed, the range of susceptibility to many of the common types of cancer may be as high as 100-fold (Harris et al. 1980, 1981). Evidence from biomolecular research supports this conviction. For example, binding levels of benzo(a)pyrene to DNA have been shown to vary from 50- to 100-fold in cultured human cells (Harris et al. 1981). This enormous variation in carcinogen interaction of human cells may be attributed to the fact that the majority of chemical carcinogens require enzymatic activation and, herein, host factors play a major role in determining variation in such enzyme capability (Pelkonen et al. 1978). Doll (1977) has postulated that the ratio of metabolic activation to deactivation of carcinogens may determine the individual's risk for cancer.

Our purpose is to discuss the role of hereditary factors in several commonly occurring cancers, namely, carcinoma of the colon, breast, and ovary.

Generalities in Cancer Genetics

Most varieties of hereditary cancer are characterized by:
(1) significantly early age of cancer onset;
(2) an excess of synchronous and metachronous cancer, and bilaterality of paired organs;
(3) specific patterns of multiple primary cancer expression in the differing hereditary cancer syndromes;

(4) occasional premonitory clinical signs [e.g., multiple adenomatous polyps in familial adenomatous polyposis (FAP), or biochemical markers such as calcitonin excess in multiple endocrine neoplasia (MEN types IIa and IIb)]; and

(5) mendelian modes of inheritance in specific hereditary syndromes.

When considering these generalities in patient assessment, it is essential to be aware of variation in the expression of each of these phenotypic features, both within and between families. Knowledge of these cardinal features of hereditary cancer will prove to be of invaluable aid in mounting highly organ-targeted surveillance and management programs. Pragmatically speaking, particularly in this era of Disease-Related Groups (DRGs), the gathering of this type of information may represent one of the most cost-effective portions of the patient's medical work-up.

Hereditary Breast Cancer

Approximately 150,900 patients in the United States in 1990 will manifest carcinoma of the breast (Silverberg and Lubera 1989). Approximately 9% (13,581) of these patients/families will have an etiology consistent with hereditary breast cancer (HBC), while an additional 20%-25% will be familial (Lynch and Lynch 1986).

Heterogeneity in HBC Syndromes

Detailed medical/genetic studies of breast cancer-prone families with meticulous verification of pathology initiated by Lynch and colleagues in the mid-1960s (Lynch and Krush 1966, 1971; Lynch et al. 1984) have been continuous and now involve several hundred kindreds in the Creighton HBC resource. These studies have aided in the comprehension of breast cancer genetics and have disclosed various features of HBC's natural history (Lynch et al. 1972), including improved survival of HBC patients when compared with those suffering from its sporadic counterpart (Lynch et al. 1984). They have also served to delineate certain differences between HBC and sporadic breast cancer and have indicated phenotypic heterogeneity within HBC subsets (Fig. 1). This heterogeneity involves age of onset (Lynch et al. 1988a,b,c) and the occurrence of associated tumors (Lynch et al. 1972, 1978a,b). It is unknown whether all or most phenotypic variants of HBC involve an abnormality at one locus (possibly with a variety of defective alleles) or whether several loci are involved, one in each etiologic subset of families.

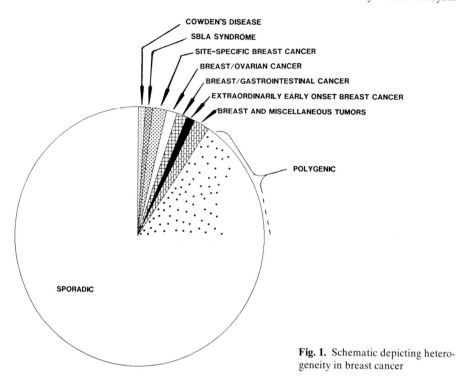

Fig. 1. Schematic depicting heterogeneity in breast cancer

Markedly Early Onset HBC Pedigrees

We have identified a subset of HBC families wherein remarkably early onset of breast cancer occurred (Fig. 2). This study involved the relationship between age of onset of breast cancer in 328 breast cancer probands (consecutively ascertained patients from our oncology clinic) and breast cancer incidence and age of onset in their female relatives. We found that a family history of early onset breast cancer was associated with a higher risk of early onset breast cancer. A family history of early onset breast cancer occurred more frequently among young (< 40) breast cancer probands than among older (> 40) breast cancer probands ($p < 0.001$; odds ratio (OR) = 23). This relationship was particularly evident when the analysis was restricted to the hereditary breast cancer probands ($p < 0.001$; OR = 33). We also observed a positive family history of breast cancer (any age) more frequently in young than in older breast cancer probands ($p < 0.001$; OR = 2.9) (Lynch et al. 1988b).

Extremely early age of breast cancer onset appears to be an additional example of heterogeneity in HBC and may represent the first account (Fig. 2) of this remarkable subset (Lynch et al. 1988a,b,c). We have also recognized breast-cancer-prone families which are characterized by late (> age 60) age of onset (Lynch 1989, unpublished data).

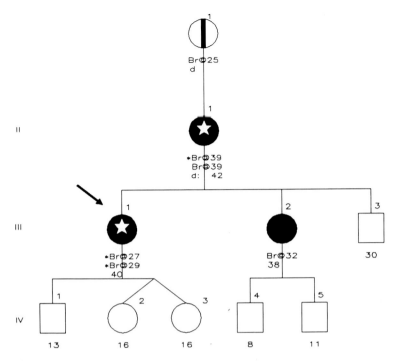

Fig. 2. Family B. Patient (*arrow*) with bilateral breast cancer, with first lesion at age 27, and each primary relative showing remarkably early onset through three generations (reproduced by permission from Lynch et al. 1988a)

Surveillance/Management

Patients who are at 50% risk for HBC (first degree relative of HBC affected) require intensive surveillance which differs significantly from standard recommendations in that these strategies must be responsive to the natural history of HBC. Thus, in the midteens, we recommend that the physician initiate an educational program which should cover genetic risk and those salient facets of HBC's natural history which will be useful to these-at-risk patients. Women should be taught breast self-examination (BSE) by their late teens and should be able to demonstrate proficiency in the performance of this procedure. They require semiannual physician examination. Mammography should be initiated by age 25, performed biennially through age 35, and annually thereafter. In those families with extraodinary early onset, particularly where it occurs in the 20s and early 30s, we recommended that mammography be initiated at age 20 years and be repeated annually. While difficulty may be encountered in the interpretation of mammograms in these young women due to increased density of the breast, recent evidence indicates that grouped microcalcifications, as sole indicators of malignancy, occur with greater frequency and can be detected in the presence of increased parenchymal density (Herman et al. 1988; Meyer et al. 1983; Sickles

1986). Attention must also be given to cancers of other anatomic sites that may be integral to HBC syndrome diagnosis, such as carcinoma of the ovary in the breast/ovarian carcinoma syndrome.

Prophylactic Therapy

The most common setting for which prophylactic therapy must be considered is a patient from a known HBC family who presents with an ipsilateral breast cancer. The autosomal dominant inheritance pattern of HBC dictates that 50% of women in the direct genetic lineage of any given HBC family (a patient with mother, sister, or daughter affected with breast cancer) are at risk of carrying the deleterious cancer-prone genotype. The development of an ipsilateral breast cancer in the HBC setting suggests that this patient does indeed harbor the cancer-prone genome (obligate gene carrier). On the other hand, the prevalence of breast cancer in the general population is great enough that there is the possibility that a random event occurred and the patient is not actually affected by HBC. Nevertheless, from a practical standpoint, this patient should have recommendations made based on the assumption that she has a 100% lifetime risk for contralateral breast cancer. This is because at the present time there is no biological or molecular genetic marker available for the diagnosis of HBC. In fact, Harris et al. (1978) showed that 46% of HBC patients with an ipsilateral malignancy will develop cancer of the contralateral breast within 20 years. The risk for breast cancer after 20 years was 5.9% per year. Because one must depend solely on the family history to confirm the presence of HBC, the HBC kindred as a whole is best served by the bilateral treatment recommendation.

The procedure of choice for patients who present with unilateral malignancies, wherein the initial cancer is of low stage with reasonable assurance of long-term survival, is bilateral total mastectomy with axillary lymph node dissection on the ipsilateral side. This procedure eliminates most tissue at risk for cancer and at tne same time allows for adequate staging of the primary tumor. Subcutaneous mastectomy for the contralateral breast should be discourage. There is increasing evidence that 10%-30% of breast tissue remains after this procedure (Goodnight et al. 1984). Case reports are now appearing describing primary breast cancer developing in residual breast tissue after the procedure. This is unacceptable in this high-risk group of patients (Eldar et al. 1984; Humphrey 1983).

Another important group of patients are those from HBC families who are unaffected but who are at 50% genetic risk and who may inquire about prophylactic bilateral mastectomy. The autosomal dominant inheritance pattern of HBC dictates that only 50% of the women in the direct genetic lineage of an HBC family will actually be harboring the deleterious gene. Thus, for patients who do not have breast cancer but have presented because they are aware that they are members of an HBC kindred, we recommend careful surveillance (see previous section). However, there is an occasional patient in whom a recommendation for prophylactic bilateral mastectomy is made. Severe cancer phobia is the most common indication especially when compounded by significant benign breast disease (particularly proliferative disease with atypia), breasts that are difficult to examine by patient and physician, history of multiple breast biopsies, breasts that are difficult to evaluate mammographically, and/or patient compliance problems. The candidates for prophylactic bilateral mastectomy should be carefully counselled, their emotional status should be evaluated, and ideally their spouses should share in the decision. An opinion from a clinical geneticist may be in the best interest of the patient. Finally, augmentation mammoplasty, given the attendant greater difficulty for diagnosis of early breast cancer (Silverstein et al. 1988), should be discouraged in patients at risk for HBC.

Molecular Genetics in Breast Cancer

Callahan and Campbell (1989) have reviewed molecular research on human breast cancer. Much of this interest has been promulgated by investigations in mice infected with the mouse mammary tumor virus, as well as in certain strains of transgenic mice with an activated oncogene, all of which have provided evidence that multiple mutations may be responsible for initiation and progression of breast cancer in these rodent models. The molecular approach in humans has been abetted by the availability of recombinant DNA probes. These enable investigators to detect proto-oncogenes, growth factor receptor genes, and restriction fragment length polymorphisms (RFLPs), which facilitate the identification of frequently occurring mutations in primary breast tumor DNA in humans. There is interest in whether specific mutations are closely associated with differing clinical parameters such as prognosis. Herein, eight mutations have been identified. These include amplification of c-*myc*, c-*erb*B2, and *int-2*, in addition to loss of heterozygosity on chromosomes 1q, 3p, 11p, 13q, and 17p. This loss of heterozygosity is believed to unmask recessive mutations of tumor suppressor genes, and risk of relapse and/or poor survival have been shown to be associated with either c-*myc*, c-*erb*B2, or *int-2*. Nevertheless, in spite of this prodigious activity, particularly with respect to the role of these mutations as prognostic indicators, the subject remains controversial and will require continued investigation.

Ali et al. (1989) described biomolecular findings from a study of 84 informative (heterozygous) primary breast tumors. Of these, 30% showed losses of heterozygosity on chromosome 3. It is of interest that the loss of heterozygosity of genes on the short arm of chromosome 3 (3p) in these human breast cancers occurred in a region wherein other malignancies, including carcinoma of the lung, renal cell carcinoma, and Von Hippel-Lindau's disease, characterized by cerebellar hemangioblastoma, renal cell carcinoma, and cancer of other anatomic sites are known to occur. It therefore appears that this specific region on chromosome 3 plays an important role in the etiology of several cancers, including carcinoma of the breast. This particular region of the chromosome includes the c-*erb*A steroid (thyroid hormone receptor family c-*erb*Ab and c-*erb*A2), which may have special pertinence to cancer of the breast. These findings provide additional insight into breast carcinogenesis and provide further evidence that multiple genetic alterations are important in breast cancer.

McGuire and Naylor (1989) conclude that it would be presumptuous at this time to ascribe an etiologic role for breast cancer development with respect to any one low-frequency chromosomal loss of heterozygosity. They believe that well-focused genetic linkage studies of familial breast cancer are now required in order to identify the genes which may be causal for this disease.

Hereditary Ovarian Cancer

Increasing attention has been given to the role of genetics in the etiology of ovarian carcinoma. Indeed, a registry of familial ovarian cancer was established by Piver in 1981 at Roswell Park Memorial Institute (Piver et al. 1984). Nevertheless, less is known about the role of genetics in the total ovarian cancer burden (Piver 1987; Lynch and Kullander 1987) than in hereditary breast cancer (Lynch and Lynch 1986).

Schildkraut and Thompson (1988) evaluated data from a multicenter population-based case/control study in order to determine the degree of aggregation of ovarian carcinoma in families. Cases were comprised of 493 women aged 20–54 years who had been recently diagnosed with epithelial ovarian carcinoma. The family history of ovarian cancer was then compared with a group of 2465 controls. The results showed an odds ratio for ovarian cancer in first and second degree relatives of ovarian cancer sufferers to be 3.6 (95% confidence interval; 1.8–7.1) and 2.9 (95% confidence interval: 1.6–5.3) respectively, when compared with women lacking a family history of ovarian cancer. In a case/control study from Japan (Mori et al. 1988), it was found that women with a family history of breast, uterine (not specified as cervix or endometrial cancer), or ovarian cancer in a mother or sister showed a highly significant risk for ovarian cancer ($p < 0.001$).

The genetic relationship between carcinoma of the ovary, breast, and endometrium was examined in a population-based case/control study by Schildkraut et al. (1989). A significant genetic correlation was found between ovarian and breast cancer ($R_{12} = 0.484$). However, no significant genetic overlap was observed between carcinoma of the endometrium and either breast or ovarian cancer. These investigators concluded that their data supported the existence of a familial breast/ovarian cancer syndrome and that carcinoma of the endometrium, while known to be heritable, appeared to be genetically unrelated to cancers of the breast and ovary.

Hereditary ovarian carcinoma is exceedingly heterogeneous. For example, ovarian neoplasms have shown an association with several familial precancer disorders (Lynch et al. 1987). These include mixed gonadal dysgenesis, showing XO/XY mosaicism, with dysgerminoma or gonadoblastoma in streak gonads (Teter 1976). Peutz-Jegher's syndrome, which is associated with granulosa theca cell tumors (Christian 1971) and papillary adenocarcinoma (Humphries et al. 1966), and multiple nevoid basal cell carcinoma, which is associated with ovarian fibromas (Lynch 1976). Ovarian fibromas have also been described on a site-specific basis in the absence of the multiple nevoid basal cell carcinoma syndrome as reported by Dumont-Herskowitz et al. (1978). Ovarian carcinoma also is an integral lesion in Lynch syndrome II (Lynch and Lynch 1979; Lynch et al. 1985a).

In our experience, the most frequently occurring hereditary expression of ovarian cancer is found in the hereditary breast/ovarian cancer syndrome (Lynch et al. 1978; Lynch and Kullander 1987; Lynch et al. 1990a).

Management

Surveillance/management of hereditary ovarian cancer is exceedingly difficult since there are no premonitory clinical signs or biomarkers of cancer suscep-tibility. In patients who are at risk for any form of hereditary cancer, inclusive of carcinoma of the ovary, we recommend an educational program with genetic counselling, to be initiated by the late teens or early 20s. The natural history of the disease should be discussed in detail, in context with the classification of genetic risk. In the case of hereditary ovarian cancer, bimanual pelvic examination should be initiated when the patient becomes sexually active and/or by age 25. Concurrent with this, we recommend ovarian ultrasound (vaginal probe ovarian ultrasound is preferred). These procedures should be done each year. We are also evaluating serum CA-125. However, it is important to note that there are no solid data available for the sensitivity or specificity of these recommended surveillance procedures.

When that patient who is at 50% risk for ovarian cancer has completed her family, and with careful consultation with her spouse or significant other, total abdominal hysterectomy with bilateral salpingo-oophorectomy should be con-sidered. It is important to advise these patients of the possible need for estrogen replacement given menopausal symptoms and the risk of developing osteopo-rosis. The patient should also be advised that there is no guarantee that this prophylactic surgery will eliminate the risk for ovarian carcinoma, given the evidence of intra-abdominal mesothelial adenocarcinoma consonant with ova-rian cancer. This problem has been documented in a fraction of patients who have undergone prophylactic oophorectomy where careful histologic examination indicated apparently normal ovaries (Tobacman et al. 1982, Lynch et al. 1986a).

Hereditary Colorectal Cancer

Hereditary colorectal cancer is broadly classified into familal adenomatous polyposis (FAP) and hereditary nonpolyposis colorectal cancer (HNPCC) (Lynch and Lynch 1985). A third putative category, hereditary discrete color-ectal polyps and cancer, has been recently described (Burt et al. 1985; Cannon-Albright et al. 1989). The flat adenoma syndrome may even represent a fourth category (Lynch et al. 1988d). We shall only consider HNPCC in this chapter.

In recent years it has become evident that a predisposition to colorectal cancer is transmitted by simple autosomal dominant inheritance in some families in the absence of diffuse polyposis of the colon (Lynch and Lynch 1985; Lynch 1986; Lovett 1976). This is not the same as the increased empiric risk of colon cancer attributed to the presence of "one or more first degree relatives with colon cancer" (Bonelli et al. 1988; Kune et al. 1987). Rather, it connotes the presence of a discrete disorder with definite clinical features. This problem merits greater investigation as it may have important implications for understanding the etiology of common colon cancer.

Definition of HNPCC (Lynch Syndromes I and II)

HNPCC is subdivided into Lynch syndromes I and II. Lynch syndrome I is characterized by an autosomal dominantly inherited predisposition to site-specific colorectal cancer with proximal predominance, an excess of synchronous and metachronous cancer of the colorectum, and early age of cancer onset in the absence of diffuse polyposis. Lynch syndrome II contains all of the colorectal cancer features of Lynch I but in addition shows an excess of extracolonic primary cancer, particularly carcinoma of the endometrium and ovary (Lynch and Lynch 1979). More recently, attention has been given to additional cancer types, namely, stomach (Cristofaro et al. 1987), small bowel (Lynch et al. 1989), pancreas (Lynch et al. 1985b), and urological (Lynch et al. 1990).

Incidence

HNPCC is now recognized as constituting a highly significant fraction of the overall colorectal cancer burden (Lynch and Lynch 1985). Based on anecdotal information during more than two decades of study, Lynch et al. predicted that 5%-6% of *all* cases of colorectal cancer would fulfill the criteria for HNPCC. Mecklin's most recent estimate (1987) of the frequency of HNPCC involved the study of all colorectal cancer patients ($n = 468$) who were diagnosed in one Finnish county (0.25 million inhabitants) during the period 1970–1979. It is of interest that HNPCC emerged as the most common risk factor for colonic cancer, involving 4%-6% of all colorectal cancer patients identified in this study. In contrast, the frequency of FAP and ulcerative colitis was only 0.2% and 0.6%, respectively.

Since HNPCC lacks distinguishing physical signs and/or biomarker(s) which clearly aid in the depiction of genetic risk status, one must rely heavily on extended pedigree studies for its recognition. These facts led Mecklin to conclude that the observed frequency of 4%-6% for HNPCC may represent an underestimate (Mecklin 1987).

Minimal Diagnostic Clues: Implications for Surveillance and Management

The clinician is frequently faced with the vexing question: "What are the minimal criteria for diagnosis of the Lynch syndromes?" Unfortunately, in the absence of specific biomarkers and/or premonitory stigmata, this cannot be answered with precision. However, our group has published accounts of many clinical examples in which cumulative knowledge of the patient's cancer family history can lead to confidence in the diagnosis of the Lynch syndromes (Lynch et al. 1988e; Lynch and Lynch 1985). For instance, colon cancer in a young patient who lacks multiple colonic polyps is the first clue. If the lesion is proximal to the splenic flexure, the index of suspicion should be raised. If, on review of the family history, a high proportion of colon cancer (especially proximal location) or endometrial cancer is seen, particularly early onset, in a pattern suggestive of autosomal dominance, the clinician can be more comfortable with the diagnosis of the Lynch syndromes. The diagnosis will be strengthened further by a history of high incidence of synchronous and/or metachronous colon cancers and/or multiple primary cancer of certain extracolonic sites.

In determining when to begin a surveillance program, age of onset and natural history of the colon carcinomas must necessarily be considered. Fortunately, in this instance, there are reasonably good data on this subject from several sources. Meckling (1987) has estimated the penetrance of the gene as being nearly complete, which is in accord with our own observations (Bailey-Wilson et al. 1986). The youngest patient with colon carcinoma from a presumed Lynch syndrome family is a 14-year-old female (Aiges et al. 1979). The onset of colorectal carcinoma appears to occur 15–20 years earlier than in the general population (Lynch and Lynch 1985). In the study of Swaroop et al. (1987), patients with multiple primary malignant tumors had diagnosis of the first cancer at a mean of 48.3 years. In Mecklin's large series from Finland (Mecklin et al. 1986), the mean age of colon cancer onset was 41 years, with a range of 19–83 years. Eighty percent of the patients were under age 50 years at the time of diagnosis of colon cancer. The mean age of colon cancer onset in our series was 45.6 years, with a range of 19–80 years of age (Lynch et al. 1988e). Age of initial diagnosis of colorectal cancer differed significantly among the 10 families which were studied. Ninety percent of the colorectal cancers had occurred by age 60 with the peak in the 40–50 age range. Using these data, we have targeted our surveillance program at the 25–60 age range (Bailey-Wilson et al. 1986; Lynch et al. 1985a).

Surveillance/Management of the Lynch Syndromes

Education and genetic counselling should begin in the mid- to late teens. Baseline colonoscopy should be initiated at age 25 and performed biannually thereafter. If colonoscopy expertise is lacking, double air contrast barium enema may be performed. Hemoccult or HemoQuant should be performed semiannually. For women, endometrial biopsy (office procedure) should be performed at age 25, with ovarian ultrasound (vaginal probe ultrasound preferred) performed annually in Lynch syndrome II. Abdominal subtotal colectomy should be performed for the presence of colorectal cancer. This is the procedure of choice because of the risk for synchronous and metachronous colorectal cancer. Prophylactic hysterectomy and bilateral salpingo-oophorectomy may be considered at the time of colon cancer operation in selected patients at risk for Lynch syndrome II.

Cost-Effective Genetic Counselling, Education, and Psychotherapy

As an effort to provide cost-effective counselling to families, we have experimented with a dynamically oriented group therapy counselling session involving multiple family members. This is coordinated by a medical oncologist/geneticist and an informed registered nurse. We attempt to create a freewheeling question-and-answer educational and group psychotherapy session. Attention is given to a description of the natural history of the particular form of hereditary cancer, its distribution within the family, and its mode of genetic transmission. An empathetic "listening ear" is provided by the nurse and physician, thereby enabling an emotional catharsis by the participants. This exchange of feelings may not have previously been possible. In short, these high-risk, ego-involved relatives have been able to cast their "family crisis problem" into a more objective perspective. Often as a group, they are able to compare notes and identify cancer occurrences as well as genealogic relationships which heretofore may not have been known by any one individual in the kindred. In short, this approach appears to be highly effective and appreciated by these affected and at-risk-relatives. It is also cost-effective and conserves considerable professional time.

Summary and Conclusions

In conclusion knowledge of cancer genetics and its application to cancer-prone families can provide one of the most powerful and potentially cost-effective approaches for early cancer detection, prevention, and control. It is also invaluable for elucidation of etiology. The public health impact of the problem is enormous when considering that between 5% and 10% of the total cancer burden is believed to be due to primary genetic factors. In spite of the significant potential benefits to patients and their families, attention to family history of cancer is often given short shrift by physicians. Consequently, clinical expertise in identifying hereditary forms of cancer is often exceedingly limited. This may change as a result of recent advances in biomolecular genetic research wherein clinicians will be provided with added precision in their identification of patients who are destined to develop cancer.

References

Aiges HW, Kahn E, Silverberg M (1979) Adenocarcinoma of the colon in an adolescent with the Family Cancer Syndrome. J Pediat 94:632–633

Ali IU, Lidereau R, Callahan R (1989) Presence of two members of c-*erb*A receptor gene family (c-*erb*Ab and c-*erb*A2) in smallest region of somatic homozygosity on chromosome 3p21-p25 in human breast carcinoma. JNCI 81:1815–1820

Bailey-Wilson JE, Elston RC, Schuelke GS, Kimberling WJ, Albano WA, Lynch JF, Lynch HT (1986) Segregation analysis of hereditary nonpolyposis colorectal cancer. Genet Epid 3:27–38

Bishop JM (1983) Cellular oncogenes and retroviruses. Annu Rev Biochem 52:301–354

Bishop JM (1986) Oncogenes and proto-oncogenes. J Cell Phys 10 [Suppl] 4:1–5

Bonelli L, Martines H, Conio M et al. (1988) Family history of colorectal cancer as a risk factor for benign and malignant tumours of the large bowel: a case-control study. Int J Cancer 41:513–517

Burt RW, Bishop DT, Cannon LA, Dowdle MA, Lee RG, Skolnick MH (1985) Dominant inheritance of adenomatous colonic polyps and colorectal cancer. N Engl J Med 312:1540–1544

Callahan R, Campbell G (1989) Mutations in human breast cancer: an overview. JNCI 81:1780–1786

Cannon-Albright LA, Skolnick MH, Bishop DT, Lee RG, Burt RW (1988) Common inheritance of colonic adenomatous polyps and associated colorectal cancers. N Engl J Med 319:533–537

Cannon-Albright LA, Thomas TC, Bishop T, Skolnick MH, Burt RW (1989) Characteristics of familial colon cancer in a large population data base. Cancer 64:1971–1975

Christian DD (1971) Ovarian tumors: an extension of the Peutz-Jegher's syndrome. Am J Obstet Gynecol 111:529–534

Cristofaro G, Lynch HT, Caruso ML et al. (1987) New phenotypic aspects in a family with Lynch syndrome II. Cancer 57:51–58

Davenport RC (1927) A family history of choroidal sarcoma. Br J Ophthalmol 11:443–445

Doll R (1977) Strategy for detection of cancer hazards to man. Nature, 265:589–596

Dumont-Herskowitz RA, Safaii HS, Senior B (1978) Ovarian fibromata in four successive generations. J Pediat 93:621–624

Eldar S, Meguid MM, Beatty JD (1984) Cancer of the breast after prophylactic subcutaneous mastectomy. Ann Surg 184:692–693

Goodnight JE, Quagliana JM, Morton DL (1984) Failure of subcutaneous mastectomy to prevent the development of breast cancer. J Surg Oncol 26:198–201

Harris CC, Mulvihill JJ, Thorgeirsson SS, Minna JD (1980) Individual differences in cancer susceptibility. Ann Intern Med 92:809–825

Harris CC, Autrup H, Stoner G (1981) Metabolism of benzo(a)pyrene by cultured human tissues and cells. In: Gelboin HV, Ts'O PO (eds) Polycyclic hydrocarbons and cancer: chemistry, molecular biology, and environment, vol 3. Academic, New York, pp 331–345

Harris RE, Lynch HT, Guirgis HA (1978) Familial breast cancer: risk to the contralateral breast. JNCI 60:955–960

Hermann G, Janus C, Schwartz IS, Papatestas A, Hermann DG, Rabinowitz JG (1988) Occult malignant breast lesions in 114 patients: relationship to age and the presence of microcalcifications. Radiology 169:321–324

Heston WE (1974) Genetics of cancer. J Herad 65:262–272

Hogan MJ, Zimerman LE (1962) Ophthalmic pathology, an atlas and textbook, 2nd edn. Saunders, Philadelphia

Humphrey LJ (1983) Subcutaneous mastectomy is not a prophylaxis against carcinoma of the breast: opinion or knowledge? Am J Surg 145:311–312

Humphries AL, Shepherd MH, Peters HJ (1966) Peutz-Jegher's syndrome with colonic adenocarcinoma and ovarian tumor. JAMA 197:296–298

Kune GA, Kune S, Watson LF (1987) The Melbourne colorectal cancer study: characterization of patients with a family history of colorectal cancer. Dis Colon Rectum 30:600–606

Lovett E (1976) Family study in cancer of the colon and rectum. Br J Surg 63:13–18

Lynch HT (ed) (1976) Cancer genetics. Thomas, Springfield

Lynch HT, Hirayama T (eds) (1989) Genetic epidemiology of cancer. CRC, Boca Raton

Lynch HT, Krush AJ (1966) Heredity and breast cancer: implications for cancer detection. Med Times
    94:599
Lynch HT, Krush AJ (1971) Carcinoma of the breast and ovary in three families. Surg Gynecol
    133:644–648
Lynch HT, Kullander S (eds) (1987) Cancer genetics in women. CRC, Boca Raton
Lynch HT, Lynch JF (1986) Breast cancer genetics in an oncology clinic: 328 consecutive patients.
    Cancer Genet Cytogenet 22:369–372
Lynch HT Lynch PM (1979) Tumor variation in the cancer family syndrome: ovarian cancer. Am J
    Surg 138:439–442
Lynch HT, Krush AJ, Lemon HM et al. (1972) Tumor variation in families with breast cancer. JAMA
    222:1631–1635
Lynch HT, Harris RE, Guirgis HA, Maloney K, Carmody L, Lynch JF (1978a) Familial association
    of breast/ovarian cancer. Cancer 41:1543–1548
Lynch HT, Mulcahy GM, Harris RE et al. (1978b) Genetic and pathologic findings in a kindred with
    hereditary sarcoma, breast cancer, brain tumors, leukemia, lung, laryngeal, and adrenal cortical
    carcinoma. Cancer 41:2055–2067
Lynch HT, Albano WA, Heieck JJ et al. (1984) Genetics, biomarkers, and breast cancer: a review.
    Cancer Genet Cytogenet 13:43–58
Lynch HT, Kimberling WJ, Albano WA et al. (1985a) Hereditary nonpolyposis colorectal cancer,
    Parts I and II. Cancer 56 939–951
Lynch HT, Voorhees GJ, Lanspa SJ et al. (1985b) Pancreatic carcinoma and hereditary nonpolyposis
    colorectal cancer: a family study. Br J Cancer 52:271–273
Lynch HT, Bewtra C, Lynch JF (1986a) Familial ovarian carcinoma: clinical nuances. Am J Med
    81:1073–1076
Lynch HT, Bewtra C, Lynch JF (1986) Familial peritoneal ovarian carcinomatosis. Med Hypotheses
    21:171–177
Lynch HT, Kimberling WJ, Lynch JF, Brennan K (1987) Familial bladder cancer in an oncology
    clinic. Cancer Genet Cytogenet 27:161–165
Lynch HT, Conway T, Fitzgibbons RJ Jr et al. (1988a) Age of onset heterogeneity in hereditary breast
    cancer: minimal clues for diagnosis. Breast Cancer Res Treat 12:275–285
Lynch HT, Watson P, Conway T, Fitzsimmons ML, Lynch JF (1988b) Breast cancer family history
    as a risk factor for early onset breast cancer. Breast Cancer Res Treat 11:263–267
Lynch HT, Conway T, Watson P, Schreiman J, Fitzgibbons RJ Jr (1988c) Extremely early onset
    hereditary breast cancer (HBC): surveillance/management implications. Nebr Med J 73:97–100
Lynch HT, Smyrk TC, Lanspa SJ, Marcus JN, Kriegler M, Lynch JF, Appleman HD (1988d) Flat
    adenomas in a colon cancer-prone kindred. JNCI 80:278–282
Lynch HT, Watson P, Lanspa SJ et al. (1988e) Natural history of colorectal cancer in hereditary
    nonpolyposis colorectal cancer (Lynch syndromes I and II). Dis Colon Rectum 31:439–444
Lynch HT, Smyrk TC, Lynch PM, Lanspa SJ, Boman BM, Ens J, Lynch JF, Strayhorn P, Carmody
    T, Cristofaro G (1989) Adenocarcinoma of the small bowel in Lynch syndrome II. Cancer
    64:2178–2183
Lynch HT, Fitzsimmons ML, Conway TA, Bewtra C, Lynch JF (1990a) Hereditary carcinoma of the
    ovary and associated cancers: a study of two families. Gynecol Oncol 36:48–55
Lynch HT, Ens JA, Lynch JF (1990b) Lynch syndrome II and urologic manifestations. J Urol
    143:24–28
Lynch PM, Lynch HT (eds) (1985) Colon cancer genetics. Reinhold, New York
McGuire WL, Naylor SL (1989) Loss of heterozygosity in breast cancer: cause or effect? JNCI
    81:1764–1765
Mecklin JP (1987) Frequency of hereditary colorectal cancer. Gastroenterology 93:1021–1025
Mecklin JP, Sipponen P, Jarvinen HJ (1986) Histopathology of colorectal carcinomas and adenomas
    in Cancer Family Syndrome. Dis Colon Rectum 29:849–853
Meyer JE, Kopans DB, Oot R (1983) Breast cancer visualized by mammography in patients under 35.
    Radiology 147:93–94
Mori M, Harabuchi I, Miyake H, Casagrande JT, Henderson BE, Ross RK (1988) Reproductive,
    genetic, and dietary risk factors for ovarian cancer. Am J Epidemiol 128:771–777

Mulvihill JJ (1984) Clinical ecogenetics of human cancer. In: Bishop JM, Rowley JD, Graeves M (eds) Genes and cancer (UCLA symposia on molecular and cellular biology, new series, vol 17). Liss, New York, pp 19–36

Norris W (1920) A case of fungoid disease. Edinb Med Surg J 16:562–565

Parsons JH (ed) (1905) The pathology of the eye, vol 2. Putnam, New York, pp 496–497

Pelkonen O, Boobis AR, Nebert DW (1978) Genetic differences in the binding of reactive carcinogenic metabolites to DNA. Carcinogenesis 3:383–400

Piver MS (ed) (1987) Ovarian malignancies: diagnostic and therapeutic advances, 2nd edn. Churchill-Livingstone, Edinburgh

Piver MS, Mettlin CJ, Tsukada Y, Nasca P, Greenwald P, McPhee ME (1984) Familial ovarian cancer registry. Obstet Gynecol 64:195–199

Schildkraut JM, Thompson WD (1988) Familial ovarian cancer: a population-based case-control study. Am J Epidemiol 128:456–466

Schildkraut JM, Risch N, Thompson WD (1989) Evaluating genetic association among ovarian, breast, and endometrial cancer: evidence for a breast/ovarian cancer relationship. Am J Hum Genet 45:521–529

Sickles EA (1986) Mammographic features of 300 consecutive nonpalpable breast cancers. AJR 146:661–663

Silcock AO (1892) Hereditary sarcoma of the eyeball in three generations. Br Med J 1:1079

Silverberg E, Lubera JA (1989) Cancer statistics 1989. Cancer 39:3–20

Silverstein MJ, Handel N, Gamagami P, Waisman JR, Gierson ED, Rosser RJ, Steyskal R, Colburn W (1988) Breast cancer in women after augmentation mammoplasty. Arch Surg 123:681–685

Swaroop VS, Winawer SJ, Kurtz RC, Lipkin M (1987) Multiple primary malignant tumors. Gastroenterology 93:779–783

Teter J (1976) Cytogenetics with reference to gonadoblastoma and to gonocytomas. In: Lynch HT (ed) Cancer genetics. Thomas, Springfield, 146–184

Tobacman JK, Greene MH, Tucker MA, Costa J, Kase R, Frameni JF Jr (1982) Intra-abdominal carcinomatosis after prophylactic oophorectomy in ovarian cancer-prone families. Lancet II:795–797

Tucker DP, Steinberg AG, Cogan DG (1975) Frequency of genetic transmission of sporadic retinoblastoma. Arch Ophthalmol 57:532–535

Pitfalls and Prospects
in Genetic Epidemiology of Cancer

N.E. MORTON

A generation ago, Neel (1955) wrote *On some pitfalls in developing an adequate genetic hypothesis.* His concern about homogeneity, confounding of genetic mechanisms, unsuitable controls, and unique aspects of human data resonate today in genetic epidemiology, which has yet to develop the strong paradigms of cytogenetics and molecular biology. Now, even more than then, his remark that "there is no faster way to dull the edge of the beautiful mathematical tools which we now possess than to attempt to use these tools in inappropriate situations" is pertinent. My experience with some of these pitfalls has been intimate and painful. I describe them in the hope that others may avoid them.

Segregation Analysis

In classical segregation analysis the unit is the nuclear family, only the phenotypes normal and affected are distinguished, and the segregation frequency within each mating type is estimated as some combination of 0, ¼, ½ and 1, or values so close to these that simple hypotheses of incomplete penetrance, mutation, or phenocopies may reasonably be entertained (Morton 1959). This approach is seldom useful except for rare dominant or recessive genes with early onset and high penetrance, or a mixture of such genes with sporadic cases.

The development of computers at midcentury permitted extension to complex segregation analysis. Elston and Stewart (1971) generalized the unit of analysis to simple pedigrees without inbreeding loops. Potentially this gave a formulation in terms of population parameters, but the constraints of contemporary computers greatly limited that potential. In fact, only a single, diallelic locus was admitted and no allowance was made for ascertainment through affection. This biased the analysis strongly toward inference of a major locus when some other familial predisposition (not necessarily genetic) was present and even when the evidence for familiarity was merely an artefact of ascertainment through affection. Ancillary tests on transmission probabilities were introduced

CRC Genetic Epidemiology Research Group, Department of Community Medicine, University of Southampton, Southampton S09 4XY, United Kingdom

H.T. Lynch and P. Tautu (Eds.)
Recent Progress
in the Genetic Epidemiology of Cancer
© Springer-Verlag Berlin Heidelberg 1991

Table 1. Unreliability of the tau model with polygenes and skewness (from Go et al. 1978, Table 3)

Results	Number of tests	Number of errors	Error rate (%)
Fits tau criterion of major locus	130	34	26
Fits 3 criteria of major locus	130	30	23

Nominal $\alpha = 0.05$. In the absence of skewness and kurtosis, taus under polygenic inheritance are compatible with a major locus, and so the error rate is 95%. As noted by Elston (1979), the tau model "has no power to distinguish between monogenic and polygenic transmission"

of the transmission probability (tau) model to distinguish between polygenes and a major locus has led to its abandonment in recent years.

To provide a more specific test of major loci even with ascertainment through affection, Morton and MacLean (1974) implemented in nuclear families the mixed model of major locus plus multifactorial inheritance. Ascertainment was subsequently generalized through the concept of pointers as affected relatives who led to ascertainment of the nuclear family, perhaps with additional constraints on phenotypes of parents and children (Lalouel and Morton 1981). Most genetic analysis of cancer has been based on the mixed model or some approximation to it (Hasstedt 1982).

Since the tau and mixed models often give conflicting results, Lalouel et al. (1983) introduced into the POINTER program a unified model that contained both sets of parameters. This created a new situation, of surprisingly frequent occurrence, in which the likelihood of the data could be much greater for a major locus than for multifactorial inheritance, but the likelihood for nonmendelian transmission was greater still. The correct conclusion in such a case is that the analysis is in some respect faulty, perhaps by misspecifying ascertainment, distribution, population frequencies, numbers of alleles, numbers of loci or gene action, but this was often interpreted as evidence against a major locus.

There are three serious objections to the use of transmission probabilities. First, transmission is a surrogate for other disturbances in the data, and the biological interpretation is unclear: few investigators would be prepared to invoke meiotic drive for a trait of unknown inheritance. Secondly, the model is formulated in such a way that if f_i is the frequency of the ith genotype, where $i = 1, 2, 3$ for AA, Aa, aa, then in the next generation the frequency of the abnormal allele (a) is

$$q' = 1 - \sum_{i=1}^{3} f_i \tau_i$$

Under Hardy-Weinberg equilibrium this implies

$$1 - q' = (1 - q)^2 \tau_i + 2q(1 - q) \tau_2 + q^2 \tau_3$$

where q is the abnormal gene frequency in the preceding generation. There are only two general cases under which the gene frequency is stable: either $\tau_1 = \tau_2 = \tau_3 = 1 - q$, which implies no inheritance (as do $H = t = 0$ and $H = q = 0$), or the mendelian case $\tau_1 = 1, \tau_2 = \frac{1}{2}, \tau_3 = 0$. Other transmission probabilities lead to changing gene frequencies. To which generation then do the population parameters apply, and how can this unstable situation be interpreted? No satisfactory answer to these questions has been provided by advocates of transmission probabilities. However, there have been instances when apparent nonmendelian transmission was induced by failure of distributional or ascertainment assumptions (Morton 1984; Demenais et al. 1986a). This muted criticism: transmission probabilities could not be relied upon to detect disturbances in the data and their interpretation was difficult except when a gross discrepancy was deliberately induced, but occasionally they were of some use.

Transmission probabilities passed from chronic to acute irritation at Genetic Analysis Workshop IV. In the first population-based sample of breast cancer submitted to complex segregation analysis (Jacobsen 1946), Williams and Anderson (1984) had inferred a rare dominant gene or genes as the only significant cause of familial aggregation. In conformity with general usage they had tested for departure of τ_2 from ½ and found no significant deviation. However, in the same data Demenais et al. (1986a) estimated all the transmission probabilities and obtained a striking increase in likelihood. They concluded that "a dominant gene could not account for the familial distribution of breast cancer in the entire sample". This appeared to be a serious criticism, since no other disturbance was clearly significant and dominant genes have been inferred from clinical case histories, selected pedigrees and subsequent population samples.

We have investigated this problem extensively and have discovered a third difficulty with transmission probabilities (Iselius et al., submitted). As implemented in POINTER, they are correctly programmed only for families under complete selection, without pointers or mutation. This is most easily demonstrated by obtaining the likelihood under a mendelian hypothesis and then disturbing the transmission probabilities to any extent and in any direction. When they are estimated with the other parameters taking their values under mendelian inheritance, the mendelian transmission probabilities are never recovered and the likelihood goes to a higher maximum, largely due to the deviation of τ_1 from 1, except when the sample is restricted to families under complete selection, without pointers or mutation. In all other cases the results are invalid. While it is embarrassing to find such an error in a program one has trusted, albeit without estimating τ_1, it is gratifying to find that rare dominant genes in breast cancer are supported, and this model may reasonably be used in the search for linkage.

Although other studies are in qualitative agreement, there are many quantitative differences associated with violations of the mixed model as currently implemented. Elston and Bailey-Wilson (1986) criticized the heterogeneity tests of Williams and Anderson (1984) as of unknown power (how many tests of multiparameter hypotheses have known power?) and then introduced an ad hoc test of unknown power and ambiguous interpretation which in the event was nonsignificant. Cannings and Thompson (1977) derived an ascertainment measure under single selection. An attempted generalization to "ascertainment events" was shown by Boehnke and Greenberg (1984) to be in serious error, but used by Cannon et al. (1986) for single pedigrees of breast cancer under multiplex selection and a model in which risks rather than odds were taken to be proportional, leading to underestimation of sporadic cases and exaggeration of lifetime risks for gene carriers.

Current segregation analysis assumes that the gene frequency is constant at all ages, whereas any gene causing specific mortality must decrease with age. The correct morbid risk for affection in a random individual who at last observation was in age class j is

$$R_j = \frac{I_j - M_{j-1}}{1 - M_{j-1}}$$

where I_j is the cumulative incidence to the midpoint of the interval and M_{j-1} is the cumulative mortality to the end of the preceding interval. All published analyses have neglected mortality, and many of them have introduced age at onset into morbid risk. This exaggerates evidence for a major locus and in extreme cases simulates nonmendelian transmission. Age of onset and other measures of severity should be incorporated into segregation analysis, but the mixed model as implemented in POINTER does not allow this. A corollary is that probands are assumed to be drawn at random from the severity distribution, and any selection of probands (for example, as premenopausal or bilateral) is a violation of the current model. With all these sources of error, the estimates in Table 2 must be taken as merely suggestive — adequate for a linkage test, but unsatisfactory for genetic counselling.

Clearly the limitation of current segregation analysis must be removed. What are the prospects? The mixed model has all the mathematical difficulties of multivariate probit analysis, and so genetic epidemiologists are following in the footsteps of statisticians by turning to log-linear models. Unfortunately, the first application has been to regressive models, which condition a person's phenotype on phenotypes of antecedents, perhaps after allowing for major loci (Bonney 1984). Class A regressive models use only parental phenotypes and therefore

Table 2. Segregation analysis of breast cancer

Authors	Dominant model ($d = 1$)		Lifetime penetrance	Comment
	displacement	gene frequency		
Bishop and Gardner (1980)	1.9	0.0056	0.84	Ascertainment and prevalence not specified
Go et al. (1983)	?	?	> 0.9	Ascertainment and prevalence ignored
Williams and Anderson (1984)	1.7	0.0076	0.57	Possible enrichment of premenopausal onset
Goldstein et al. (1987)	2.8	0.0014	?	Bilateral probands, onset substituted for current age
Newman et al. (1988)	2.3	0.0006	0.82	Premenopausal probands, onset substituted for current age
Bishop et al. (1988)	?	0.0002	~0.84	"Ascertainment event" correction of high-risk pedigrees

misinterpret sibling environment as dominance of a major gene. In the special case of complete selection, multivariate normality and phenotypes known for both parents, the class D regressive model reduces to the mixed model. Generalization of regressive models to qualitative traits or untested parents does not correspond to any genetic model and the few applications have been discouraging. For example, Bonney et al. (1986) converted sibling recurrence into a claim that chronic atrophic gastritis in the Narino region of Columbia is due to a recessive gene with a frequency of 0.78. Such results raise serious doubts about the capacity of log-linear regressive models to distinguish a major locus from multifactorial inheritance even if extended to include incomplete ascertainment.

Resolution of this problem begins with the fact that the multifactorial breeding value is a continuous latent variable, which log-linear models cannot accommodate. On the other hand, they can readily be extended to oligogenic hypotheses. In the two-locus model of MacLean et al. (1984) multifactorial inheritance is specified by $q, q_m > 0$ and single locus inheritance by $q_m = 0$, where the gene frequency is q at the major locus and q_m at the modifier locus. A wide range of parent-offspring and sib correlations can be represented by $q_m = 0.5$, especially if modifier dominance d_m is not constrained to the 0, 1 interval. The pseudo-polygenic case corresponds to $q_m = d_m = 0.5$. Instead of a liability indicator, the morbid risks R in the population can be represented by a continuous state $C = \text{logit } R$ which may include risk factors such as age, parity and other situational variables that are specified without considering the affection status of the individual. If the genotypic effect is G, the variable

$$I = G + C$$

is an ousiotype that defines a specific morbid risk $e^I/(1 + e^I)$. Then information defined only for affected individuals may be expressed as severity S with specific expectation $a_s + b_s I$ and some distribution (normal, gamma, etc.) specified by two parameters which we may take to be mean and variance. For breast cancer, S should include laterality, age of onset, prognostic biomarkers, and other affective variables. Information defined only for normal individuals may be similarly expressed as diathesis D, which might include associated cancers and cystic breast disease, with specific expectation $a_D + b_D I$ and appropriate distribution specified by mean and variance. A quantitative trait ascertained through affection could enter into D and this might accurately model a rare gene, but discrimination between a polymorphism and multifactorial inheritance would probably be better for the mixed model.

Linkage

Physical and genetic locations have been determined for many proto-oncogenes that play a role in tumour progression. Curiously enough, they rarely are the site of a primary alteration leading to cancer except when transposed to controlling regions for a few critical loci like immunoglobulins, and in such cases they are usually somatic mutations. Inherited mutations are much more commonly found at loci where the normal allele suppresses tumorigenesis (anti-oncogenes) and the search for these is a major focus of genetic epidemiology. Two problems have been apparent.

First, the swept radius of a marker locus is small enough so that even a highly significant linkage test ($Z > 3$) may be a type I error. This is of course even more likely if a weaker significance level is used. Subdivision of the data into possibly more homogenous subsets, whether undertaken legitimately before a linkage analysis or heuristically afterwards, increases the likelihood of at least one type I error. Segregation parameters should either be estimated before analysing linkage or re-estimated on the null hypothesis of no linkage, otherwise the type I error will be inflated. These cautions are illustrated by false reports of breast cancer linkage to GPT (King et al. 1980) and ABO loci (Skolnick et al. 1984). Other difficulties arise with sib-pair tests based on identity by descent, which have been useful for diseases associated with the highly polymorphic HLA system. Unfortunately there is a great loss of power with less polymorphic loci, especially if parents are not tested (Weeks and Lange 1988). Affection status of parents is used effectively only under a genetic model (Morton 1983). The best sib-pair test for a rare dominant is poor for a rare recessive, and vice versa. Recombination values and map distance cannot be estimated, except on untested assumptions, since there is no rigorous discrimination among recombination, heterogeneity, incomplete penetrance, mistyping and other misspecification of the model. In short, there is no example where a sib-pair test has revealed something that conventional linkage tests did not do better. The weakness of sib-pair tests should not be taken as an argument against preferential sampling of affected relatives and their parents, which under recessivity or low penetrance may be a cost-effective strategy. However, the merit of sib-pair methods for analysis of such data is dubious.

Once linkage has been detected, localization depends upon standard maps derived largely from the CEPH consortium. The comprehensive map attempts to include all syntenic loci, while the skeletal map is limited to loci with well-supported order (Morton and Collins, 1990). The resolution of the skeletal map approaches 5 cM in males and 10 cM in females, which is inadequate both for the Human Genome Project, which calls for a standard map at 1 cM resolution, and for precise localization of disease genes. In practice, therefore, disease loci will be mapped in relation to loci in the comprehensive map within regions defined by the closest flanking skeletal loci, and the same strategy would be used to connect sequence tagged sites (Olson et al. 1989).

Association

Selection of controls is as much a problem today as when Neel (1955) stigmatized selection bias. The problem is particularly acute in pedigree studies where there may be a real difference among cohorts in morbid risks or an apparent difference due to over- or under-diagnosis of affection among relatives of second or higher degree, simulating gene interaction. A sensitivity analysis is required to verify that the conclusions are robust to reasonable changes in control frequencies.

Association studies present similar problems. Often cases and controls are not randomized or matched for ethnic group or other relevant variables, and the interviewers, clinicians and laboratory workers who collect critical data are not blind to the distinction. The claim of an increased frequency of rare HRAS alleles among cancer patients of various types (Krontiris et al. 1985) has received such inconsistent support as to be seriously compromised, and all attempts to detect close linkage of a tumour suppressor to HRAS have failed (Hall et al. 1989). Loss of heterozygosity, amplification, mutation and other oncogene alterations are associated with tumour progression and thus may be of prognostic value in patients, if not their families.

Envoi

Genetic epidemiology is entering a new era in which it will work with established loci, a dense linkage map and tested methods. However, this inviting prospect is not without danger. We have entertained unjustified claims of major loci, linkage and association. Increasingly we are using computer programs whose assumptions are nowhere clearly stated (Lange et al. 1988; Konigsberg et al. 1989). We rely on Genetic Analysis Workshops to correct some of these deficiencies, but the number, brevity and diversity of their contributions frustrate synthesis and reflect failure to pose (and therefore to answer) any specific questions. The discipline of genetic epidemiology is overshadowed by an enormous congregation of human geneticists, and ties with epidemiology are weak. When the Genetics Society of America failed to accommodate specialized groups, it split into sections dealing with yeast, *Drosophila*, and evolutionary genetics. Perhaps the much larger American Society of Human Genetics is approaching its diaspora. In Europe, specialized groups form without trauma, as they once did in America. Whether or not this happens to genetic epidemiology, we must find a middle ground between loss of identity in a crowd and lack of stimulation in a cell. I suspect the solution may lie in symposia such as this.

References

Bishop DT, Gardner EJ (1980) Analysis of the genetic predisposition to cancer in individual pedigrees. In: Cairns J, Lyon JL, Skolnick M Cancer incidence in defined populations. Banbury report 4. Cold Spring Harbor, New York, pp 389–406
Bishop DT, Cannon-Albright L, McLellan T, Gardner EJ, Skolnick MH (1988) Segregation and linkage analysis of nine Utah breast cancer pedigrees. Genet Epidemiol 5:151–170
Boehnke M, Greenberg DA (1984) The effects of conditioning on probands to correct for multiple ascertainment. Am J Hum Genet 36:1298–1308

Bonney GE (1984) On the statistical determination of major gene mechanisms in continuous human traits: regressive models. Am J Med Genet 18:731–749

Bonney GE, Elson RC, Correa P, Haenszel W, Zavala DE, Zarama G, Collazos T, Cuello C (1986) Genetic etiology of gastric carcinoma. I. Chronic atrophic gastritis. Genet Epidemiol 3:213–224

Cannings C, Thompson EA (1977) Ascertainment in the sequential sampling of pedigrees. Clin Genet 12:208–212

Cannon LA, Bishop DT, Skolnick MH (1986) Segregation and linkage analysis of breast cancer in the Dutch and Utah families. Genet Epidemiol (suppl) 1:43–48

Demenais F, Lathrop M, Lalouel J-M (1986a) Robustness and power of the unified model in the analysis of quantitative measurements. Am J Hum Genet 38:228–234

Demenais F, Martinez M, Bonaïti-Pellié C, Clerget-Darpoux F, Feingold N (1986b) Segregation analysis of the Jacobsen data. Genet Epidemiol (suppl) 1:49–54

Elston RC (1979) Major locus analysis for quantitative traits. Am J Hum Genet 31:655–661

Elston RC, Bailey-Wilson JE (1986) Critique of a published analysis of the Jacobsen data. Genet Epidemiol (suppl) 1:55–59

Elston RC, Stewart J (1971) A general model for the genetic analysis of pedigree data. Hum Hered 21:523–542

Go RCP, Elston RC, Kaplan EM (1978) Efficiency and robustness of pedigree segregation analysis. Am J Hum Genet 30:28–37

Go RCP, King M-C, Bailey-Wilson J, Elston RC, Lynch HT (1983) Genetic epidemiology of breast cancer and associated cancers in high-risk families. I. Segregation analysis. JNCI 71:455–461

Goldstein AM, Haile RWC, Marazita ML, Paganini-Hill A (1987) A genetic epidemiologic investigation of breast cancer in families with bilateral breast cancer. I. Segregation analysis. JNCI 78:911–918

Hall MJ, Zuppan PJ, Anderson LA, Huey B, Carter C, King M-C (1989) Oncogenes and human breast cancer. Am J Hum Genet 44:577–584

Hasstedt SJ (1982) A mixed model likelihood approximation on large pedigrees. Comput Biomed Res 15:295–307

Jacobsen O (1946) Heredity and breast cancer. Lewis, London

King M-C, Go RCP, Elston RC, Lynch HT, Petrakis NL (1980) Allele increasing susceptibility to human breast cancer may be linked to the glutamate-pyruvate transaminase locus. Science 208:406–408

Konigsberg LW, Kammerer CM, MacCluer JW (1989) Segregation analysis of quantitative traits in nuclear families: comparison of three program packages. Genet Epidemiol 6:713–726

Krontiris TG, DiMartino NA, Colb M, Parkinson DR (1985) Unique allelic restriction fragments of the human Ha-ras locus in leukocyte and tumour DNAs of cancer patients. Nature 36:460–465

Lalouel J-M, Morton NE (1981) Complex segregation analysis with pointers. Hum Hered 31:312–321

Lalouel J-M, Morton NE, Elston RC (1983) A unified model for complex segregation analysis. Am J Hum Genet 35:816–826

Lange K, Weeks D, Boehnke M (1988) Letter to the editor. Programs for pedigree analysis: MENDEL, FISHER, and dGENE. Genet Epidemiol 5:471–472

MacLean CJ, Morton NE, Yee S (1984) Combined analysis of genetic segregation and linkage under an oligogenic model. Comput Biomed Res 17:471–480

Morton NE (1959) Genetic tests under incomplete ascertainment. Am J Hum Genet 11:1–16

Morton NE (1983) An exact linkage test for multiple case families. Hum Hered 33:244–249

Morton NE (1984) Trials of segregation analysis by deterministic and Monte Carlo simulation. In: Chakravarti A (ed) Human population genetics. Van Nostrand Reinhold, New York, pp 83–107

Morton NE, Collins A (1990) Standard maps of chromosome 10. Ann Hum Genet 54:235–251

Morton NE, MacLean CJ (1974) Analysis of family resemblance. III. Complex segregation of quantitative traits. Am J Hum Genet 26:489–503

Neel JV (1955) On some pitfalls in developing an adequate genetic hypothesis. Am J Hum Genet 7:1–14

Newman B, Austin MA, Lee M, King M-C (1988) Inheritance of human breast cancer: evidence for autosomal dominant transmission in high-risk families. Proc Natl Acad Sci USA 85:3044–3048

Olson M, Hood L, Cantor C, Botstein D (1989) A common language for physical mapping of the human genome. Science 24:1434–1435

Skolnick MH, Thompson EA, Bishop DT, Cannon LA (1984) Possible linkage of a breast cancer susceptibility locus to the ABO locus: sensitivity of lod scores to a single new recombinant observation. Genet Epidemiol 1:363–374

Weeks DE, Lange K (1988) The affected-pedigree-member method of linkage analysis. Am J Hum Genet 42:315–326

Williams WE, Anderson DE (1984) Genetic epidemiology of breast cancer: segregation analysis of 200 Danish pedigrees. Genet Epidemiol 1:7–20

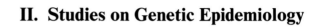

II. Studies on Genetic Epidemiology

Familial Susceptibility to Breast Cancer

N. Andrieu[1], F. Clavel[1], and F. Demenais[2]

Introduction

Familial concentrations of breast cancer, first described over 100 years ago (Broca 1866), may be due either to chance or to environmental factors common to members of the same family. They may also result from genetic susceptibility to the disease.

Familial concentrations have been observed in all ethnic groups, even in regions with low breast cancer incidence. The observed differences in breast cancer incidence among different ethnic groups of the same country could be explained by genetic factors (Petrakis et al. 1982). Even though the increase in the risk of breast cancer observed over one or two generations in populations migrating from a low- to a high-risk region (Yeung 1983) might be due to a change in environmental factors, it can be assumed that this change favors the expression of certain genetic factors.

In epidemiological studies (Kelsey 1979), the risk of breast cancer was found to increase for women who had a first degree relative with this disease (relative risk = 1.5–3). This increased risk is found in all epidemiological studies.

Therefore, susceptibility to this type of cancer appears to result from complex interactions between genetic and environmental factors. One possible approach for a better understanding of the genetic mechanisms involved is segregation analysis. Its main aim is to search for the presence of a major gene among the set of factors determining the disease, by testing different genetic hypotheses which might explain its familial transmission.

Attempts to Identify a Major Gene

The main studies (Table 1) which have used segregation analysis in an attempt to identify a gene controlling susceptibility to breast cancer are reviewed hereafter.

Analyses were performed either on genealogies usually ascertained primarily for linkage analysis (i.e., for clusters of breast cancer cases) or on nuclear families (mothers, sisters).

[1] Unité de recherche en epidémiologie des cancers, INSERM U287, Institut Gustave Roussy, rue Camille, Desmoulins, 94805 Villejuif Cedex, France
[2] Howard University Cancer Center, 2041 Georgia Avenue, NW Washington, DC 20060, USA

H.T. Lynch and P. Tautu (Eds.)
Recent Progress
in the Genetic Epidemiology of Cancer
© Springer-Verlag Berlin Heidelberg 1991

Table 1. Attempts to identify a major gene

Mode of inheritance	Data	Origin of the data	Reference
Dominant gene	1 geneal.	USA	Hill et al. 1978
	1 geneal.	USA	Bishop and Gardner 1980
	~200 geneal.	Denmark	Williams and Anderson 1984
	1579 famil.	USA	Newman et al. 1988
No simple	18 geneal.	USA	Go et al. 1983
monogenic	~200 geneal.	Denmark	Demenais et al. 1986
inheritance	200 famil.	USA	Goldstein et al. 1987
	9 geneal.	USA	Bishop et al. 1988

geneal., genealogies; famil., nuclear families; ~, same data

Some of these studies have concluded that the pattern of breast cancer is best explained by an autosomal dominant gene. The first was made in 1978 by Hill et al. on a large genealogy of Mormons (pedigree 107). The authors confirmed the hypothesis of a dominant gene, against that of a random distribution, and concluded that there was a dominant autosomal monogenic segregation of breast cancer in this genealogy. Other authors (Bishop and Gardner 1980) reanalyzed the same genealogy using the mixed model (Morton and MacLean 1974) in an attempt to identify a multifactorial transmissible component. In agreement with Hill et al. (1978), they concluded that a major gene did exist, with heritability tending towards 0 (i.e., no multifactorial transmissible component).

In 1984, another Mormon family (pedigree 1001) was analyzed because its members included numerous cases of breast cancer. In this genealogy, susceptibility was transmitted in a dominant monogenic manner (cited by Skolnick et al. 1984).

Data collected in Denmark in 1942 and 1943 (Jacobsen 1946) concerning 200 genealogies covering four generations, made it possible to demonstrate the existence of a major gene after rejection of the sporadic and polygenic hypotheses. Williams and Anderson (1984) did not rule out the possibility that this gene might be transmitted in mendelian fashion. They concluded that a major gene for susceptibility to breast cancer segregated in these families and found that the proportion of sporadic breast cancer increased with age, reaching 87% at 80 years.

Newman et al. (1988) undertook an analysis of 1579 nuclear families (mother and sisters) of breast cancer probands diagnosed before age 55 in 1980–1982 by means of the Surveillance, Epidemiology, and End Results Program in the United States. They showed that an autosomal dominant model with a highly penetrant susceptibility allele fully explained disease clustering. But this genetic susceptibility was present in only 4% of the families. They explained disease clustering in an extended kindred at high risk of breast cancer by the same model with higher gene frequency. From these two results, they concluded that only one susceptibility gene was sufficient to explain breast cancer susceptibility in some families.

Others did not conclude in favor of a particular mode of inheritance of the disease. Eighteen Caucasian families living in the United States Midwest were investigated between 1967 and 1975. These families were selected when breast cancer occurred among at least three relatives. In 16 of the genealogies, genetic transmission seemed likely, but in the other two, the familial data were better explained by a random effect (Go et al. 1983).

Demenais et al. (1986) reanalyzed the data collected in Denmark in 1942 and 1943 by Jacobsen. They concluded that a model of dominant mendelian inheritance could not explain the transmission of breast cancer in the Danish sample. The discrepancy between their results and those of Williams and Anderson (1984) may be due to differences in testing transmission hypotheses against the transmission probability model. The rejection by Demenais et al. (1986) of the mendelian hypothesis led them to suggest that the genetic mechanism of breast cancer transmission might be heterogeneous or even more complex.

Goldstein et al. (1987) have recorded, from the cancer registry of Los Angeles County, 200 women with bilateral cancer diagnosed before 50 years of age between 1970 and 1984 and their female first degree relatives (i.e., mothers, sisters, and daughters). They assumed that pre- and postmenopausal breast cancer are two genetically distinct diseases and conducted two analyses. In one analysis, they considered that only premenopausal breast cancer cases were affected, whereas in the other, they did not make this distinction. Both analyses showed that transmission of a major gene was not sufficient to explain the distribution of the disease among the population concerned.

Bishop et al. (1988) analyzed nine pedigrees (including pedigrees 1001 and 107) chosen for a cluster of breast cancer cases. No resolution of genetic model was possible. They concluded that segregation analysis will only give meaningful estimates when a larger population base is used as the unit of analysis, rather than a small number of extended families with complex ascertainment, and that conclusions drawn from segregation analysis performed on extended genealogies ascertained for clusters of breast cancer have to be considered with some reservation.

The Causes of Heterogeneity

Breast cancer heterogeneity can be implied from clinical, histological, biochemical and epidemiological observations. A genetic heterogeneity is suggested by the results of Go et al. (1983) who found preferential associations between certain types of cancer within families (endometrial, ovarian, sarcoma, etc.) and also by the differential risk for relatives on the basis of age and laterality (unilaterality or bilaterality) of the proband's disease (Kelsey 1979). Indeed, the magnitude of the risk depends upon the menopausal status of the relative at breast cancer diagnosis (RR = 3 for premenopausal; RR = 1.5 for postmenopausal) and the laterality of that relative's cancer (RR = 5 for bilateral cancer). This risk reached a value of 9 for premenopausal and bilateral cancer. Etiologic heterogeneity for breast cancer may exist at two levels:

— heterogeneity within families, due to the occurrence of sporadic cases in families with genetic breast cancer (Bailey-Wilson et al. 1986),
— heterogeneity among families which could be defined as a consequence of susceptibility genes (still unknown) differing from family to family.

This latter genetic heterogeneity has been explored in various studies, especially by dividing a total sample into subsamples according to clinical or epidemiological criteria and reviewed hereafter (Table 2). Investigations were focused on interfamilial heterogeneity according to age, menopausal status, sex of the proband, the presence or not of other cancer sites among the proband's relatives, as well as on intrafamilial heterogeneity according to types of nuclear families constituting genealogies.

Williams and Anderson (1984) studied intrafamilial heterogeneity by comparing the four types of nuclear families constituting the Danish genealogies, but were unable to demonstrate any heterogeneity. The similarity of their estimations of heritability in maternal and paternal nuclear families, under the polygenic model, indicated that susceptibility to breast cancer is transmitted by both the paternal and the maternal sides.

Gilligan and Borecki (1986) investigated heterogeneity in the Danish genealogies according to critera related to breast cancer etiology, i.e., the proband's sex, the time of discovery of the disease (pre- or postmenopausal) and age at diagnosis (≤ 56 or > 56 years).

Demenais et al. (1986) and Andrieu et al. (1988) explored this heterogeneity in the same sample, by separating the genealogies according to the following critera: (a) types of nuclear family; (b) proband's age at diagnosis (≤ 40 and

Table 2. Search for genetic heterogeneity

Criteria	Reference	Origin of the data	Conclusions
Type of nuclear family	Williams and Anderson 1984	Denmark	Paternal and maternal transmission
Type of nuclear family	Demenais et al. 1986	Denmark	Paternal and maternal transmission
Sex of the proband	Gilligan and Borecki 1986	Denmark	Males: dominant gene Females: no single gene
Age of the proband ($\leq 56/> 56$ yrs)	Gilligan and Borecki 1986	Denmark	≤ 56 yrs: single gene > 56 yrs: no single gene
Age of the proband ($\leq 40/> 40$ yrs)	Andrieu et al. 1988	Denmark	≤ 40 yrs: no single gene > 40 yrs: no single gene
Existence or not of another cancer site	Andrieu et al. 1988	Denmark	BCA: dominant gene BCOC: no single gene
Synchronous or asynchronous tumor of the proband	Goldstein et al. 1988	USA	Syn.: recessive gene Asyn.: dominant gene

BCA, breast cancer alone in the genealogies; *BCOC*, breast cancer and others cancers in the genealogies; *Syn.*, synchronous; *Asyn.*, asynchronous

> 40); and (c) presence or absence of other cancer sites among the proband's relatives. In agreement with Williams and Anderson (1984), no intrafamilial heterogeneity was revealed. Although epidemiological studies have shown an increased risk for the female relatives of a proband diagnosed at a young age, Andrieu et al. (1988) and Gilligan et al. (1986) were unable to clearly identify distinct genetic groups. However, unlike Gilligan and Borecki (1986), Andrieu et al. (1988) found no major gene for the proband's young age group. The divergence between these results may be due to the age limits used to define each subgroup (40 and 56 years respectively). None of these authors was able to demonstrate any statistically significant heterogeneity. Nevertheless, analysis of the other subgroups suggested that the group of male probands and the group of genealogies displaying only breast cancer are genetically the most homogeneous. Indeed, Andrieu et al. (1988) have shown that mendelian segregation of a dominant gene with a small frequency ($q = 0.003$) and a high penetrance — over 50% probability of having the diseased phenotype after 50 years of age when the susceptibility gene is present — accounts well for the distribution of the disease in the genealogies with breast cancer only. Similarly, for the subgroup of male probands, Gilligan and Borecki (1986) found small frequency and high penetrance of the dominant gene.

Goldstein et al. (1987) suggested the possibility of heterogeneity based on menopausal status. They also investigated heterogeneity in their data according to interval between diagnosis of the two primary tumors in the probands (Goldstein et al. 1988). Their findings indicate that for the families in which this interval was less than one year (synchronous), the mode of inheritance was consistent with a recessive major gene model. In contrast, for the families in which this interval was at least two years (asynchronous), the mode of inheritance was consistent with a dominant major gene model. Furthermore, they classified these data with respect to menopausal status where only premenopausal breast cancer cases were considered as diseased. Heterogeneity test was significant for the single locus hypothesis but not for the mixed model. Indeed, the families of premenopausal synchronous women had breast cancer that segregated in a recessive fashion, while the mode of inheritance of the premenopausal asynchronous women resembled a dominant model.

The different conclusions drawn from the analyses of family subgroups do suggest the existence of genetic heterogeneity. Such an approach can lead to the isolation of genetically homogeneous family groups (e.g., families with breast cancer only, or families with affected males, etc.) which can be studied for linkage with various markers.

Genetic vs Environmental Effects

The relative importance of genes and environment in the etiology of breast cancer depends on the model used to explain best the transmission of susceptibility to breast cancer.

Assuming that this disease is the consequence of several successive genetic events, certain women may conceivably carry at least one of these events in their germ-line (susceptibility genes) (Knudson 1971). Thus, one possible model assumes that the presence of one or more rare genes increases the risk of breast cancer. Common and random somatic alterations would therefore induce tumorigenesis in women carrying these rare genes. This model implies that the susceptibility gene(s) would have a high penetrance and that the environment would be less important. Only a small fraction of breast cancer cases would be attributable to this type of inherited susceptibility.

A second possible model assumes that one or several common alleles would increase the sensitivity to environmental factors, such as exogenous hormones, radiation, or nutrition. The lack of exposure to these factors would explain why many women with this susceptibility do not necessarily develop breast cancer. As these susceptibility genes have low penetrance in this model, it is implied that genetic and environmental factors would be jointly responsible for the development of cancer. Many women have inherited this susceptibility, but many of them will be exempt if they are not exposed to such environmental factors. Genetic heterogeneity might exist if it is assumed that there are several genes, each of which increases sensitivity to each environmental factor (Bailey-Wilson et al. 1986).

Environment is therefore important in familial analysis. As shown by Demenais et al. (1986) and Andrieu et al. (1988), the results of segregation analysis depend on how epidemiological factors are taken into account. Consequently, it seems essential to acquire information about environmental factors at the family level. In this respect, various models have recently been developed to assess simultaneously genetic and environmental factors (Bonney 1986, Hopper and Derrick 1986).

Conclusion

The studies reviewed here have shown the probable complexity of the inheritance component of susceptibility to breast cancer. By taking into account the epidemiological factors, familial analysis would make it possible to better encompass the genetic component and to define more precisely the role of the genes concerned. For this purpose, the recent models mentioned above can be adapted to the specific problems raised by breast cancer. Moreover, the search for heterogeneity may lead to the isolation of more homogeneous subgroups. The analysis of genetic linkage with different markers within such subgroups would help to better locate the susceptibility gene(s) on the chromosome map. Guidelines for further research at the molecular level would therefore be provided.

References

Andrieu N, Demenais F, Martinez M (1988) Genetic analysis of human breast cancer: implications for family study designs. Genet Epidemiol 5:225–233

Bailey-Wilson JE, Cannon LA, King MC (1986) Genetic analysis of human breast cancer: a synthesis of contributions to GAW IV. Genet Epidemiol (suppl)1:15–35

Bishop DT, Gardner EJ (1980) Analysis of the genetic predisposition to cancer in individual pedigrees. In: Cairns J, Lyons JL, Skolnick M (eds) Cancer incidence in defined populations. Banbury Report 4. Cold Spring Harbor, New York, pp 389

Bishop DT, Cannon-Albright L, McLellan T, Gardner EJ, Skolnick MH (1988) Segregation and linkage analysis of nine Utah breast cancer pedigrees. Genet Epidemiol 5:151–169

Bonney GE (1986) Regression logistic models for familial disease and other binary traits. Biometrics 42:611–625

Broca P (1866) Traité des tumeurs. In: Anselin, Becket, Labe (eds) Des tumeurs en général. Paris

Demenais F, Martinez M, Bonaiti-Pellie C, Clerget-Darpoux F, Feingold N (1986) Segregation analysis of the Jacobsen data. Genet Epidemiol (suppl)1:49–54

Gilligan SB, Borecki IB (1986) Examination of heterogeneity in 200 Danish breast cancer pedigrees. Genet Epidemiol (suppl)1:67–72

Go RCP, King MC, Bailey-Wilson J, Elston RC, Lynch HT (1983) Genetic epidemiology of breast and associated cancers in high risk families. I. Segregation analysis. J Natl Cancer Inst 71:455–561

Goldstein AM, Haile RWC, Marazita ML, Paganini-Hill A (1987) A genetic epidemiologic investigation of breast cancer in families with bilateral breast cancer. I. Segregation analysis. J Natl Cancer Inst 78:911–918

Goldstein AM, Haile RWC, Hodge SE, Paganini-Hill A, Spence MA (1988) Possible heterogeneity in the segregation pattern of breast cancer in families with bilateral breast cancer. Genet Epidemiol 5:121–133

Hill JR, Carmelli D, Gardner EJ, Skolnick M (1978) Likelihood analysis of breast cancer predisposition in a Mormon pedigree. In: Morton NE, Chung CS (eds) Genetic epidemiology. Academic, New York, pp 304–310

Hopper JL, Derrick PL (1986) A log-linear model for binary pedigree data. Genet Epidemiol (suppl) 1:73–82

Jacobsen O (1946) Heredity in breast cancer. In: Lewis HK (ed) A genetic and clinical study of two hundred probands. London, pp 1–306

Kelsey JL (1979) A review of the epidemiology of human breast cancer. Epidemiol Rev 1:74–109

Knudson AG (1971) Mutation and cancer: statistical study of retinoblastomas. Proc Natl Acad Sci USA 68:820–823

Morton NE, MacLean CJ (1974) Analysis of family resemblance. III. Complex segregation of quantitative traits. Am J Hum Genet 26:489–503

Newman B, Austin MA, Lee M, King MC (1988) Inheritance of human breast cancer: evidence for autosomal dominant transmission in high-risk families. Proc Natl Acad Sci USA 85:3044–3048

Petrakis NL, Ernster VL, King MC (1982) Breast cancer. In: Schottenfeld D, Fraumeni JF (eds) Cancer epidemiology and prevention. Saunders, Philadelphia, p 855

Skolnick MH, Thomson EA, Bishop DT, Cannon LA (1984) Possible linkage of a breast cancer susceptibility locus to the ABO locus: sensitivity of LOD scores to a single new recombinant observation. Genet Epidemiol 1:363–373

Williams WR, Anderson DE (1984) Genetic epidemiology of breast cancer: segregation analysis of 200 Danish pedigrees. Genet Epidemiol 1:7–20

Yeung KS (1983) Epidemiology of breast cancer among chinese women in the San Francisco Bay. PhD Dissertation, University of California

Linkage Mapping of Cancer Susceptibility Genes*

D.T. Bishop[1], L.A. Cannon-Albright[2], and M.H. Skolnick[2]

Introduction

The linkage map of the human genome is particularly important for disease-mapping studies (Solomon and Bodmer 1979; Botstein et al. 1980). For instance, the location of the genes for Huntington's Disease (Gusella et al. 1983), cystic fibrosis (Tsui et al. 1985), familial adenomatous polyposis (Bodmer et al. 1987) and neurofibromatosis (Barker et al. 1987) have all been found while the rudimentary map was being developed. As of 1989, there are approximately 1500 DNA polymorphisms and an essentially complete, low-density, linkage map of the human genome (Kidd et al. 1989). While the development of the map resulted in many successful mapping studies of these rarer, monogenic syndromes, the complete linkage map has major implications for the study of complex diseases such as behavioural traits and inherited predisposition to common cancers. While the difficulties associated with mapping complex traits or diseases are more daunting, the potential impact on public health of unravelling their genetics readily warrants the change of focus.

The attraction of mapping studies of complex traits where genetic determination is less certain is that, by examining between 100 and 200 markers, we can observe inheritance of essentially the whole genome across multiple generations (Solomon and Bodmer 1979; Botstein et al. 1980). Any region consistently common to related affected individuals is a candidate region for genes that determine susceptibility to the trait of interest. If sufficient families can be found then either linkage should be found or simple homogeneous monogenic inheritance excluded. For such a study, the laboratory costs are still high but the techniques are becoming increasingly routine and automated. The pay-off is the identification of a common gene or genes that cause severe morbidity or mortality. This has medical importance for the families which possess that gene in that individual specific screening strategies could be developed, perhaps incorporating allele-specific probes. There is also scientific importance since understanding of the more penetrant genes could well give us insight into the less penetrant genes and the process of carcinogenesis in the absence of genetic

* This research was supported partially by NIH awards CA-28854 and CA-36362
[1] Genetic Epidemiology Laboratory, Imperial Cancer Research Fund, Leeds, United Kingdom
[2] Department of Medicine, University of Utah School of Medicine, Salt Lake City, UT, USA

H.T. Lynch and P. Tautu (Eds.)
Recent Progress
in the Genetic Epidemiology of Cancer
© Springer-Verlag Berlin Heidelberg 1991

susceptibility. This has been the case, for instance, with the chromosome 5q locus for familial adenomatous polyposis which is now known to be deleted in the majority of colorectal malignancies (Bodmer 1990; Solomon et al. 1987; Ashton-Rickardt et al. 1989).

For this discussion, a complex disease is a trait which is known to show familial aggregation but whose pattern of affection within pedigrees does not provide clear evidence for single-locus mendelian inheritance. For cancer, we think of these loci as determining susceptibility to cancer since carriers are much more likely but not assured to develop the cancer. These traits are characterized by partial penetrance, varying expression within the families and often environmental factors which on a population level are thought to be important. Such environmental factors often represent an alternative explanation for the observed familial aggregation. However, knowledge of a significant environmental risk factor does not necessarily negate a genetic predisposition since the carcinogenic process may logically involve genetic and environmental factors acting together or independently at different points in time. Mapping provides the possibility of identifying the significant genetic factors in this sequence.

In this discussion, we present a review of current thoughts and practice in the search for genes related to complex diseases; we will concentrate on cancer studies although most of these concepts are valid for other mapping studies. We will discuss issues related to determining the appropriate sampling unit and methods of analysis. We will emphasize the importance of a detailed and careful understanding of the family patterns of disease expression prior to submitting DNA to molecular markers or even a family member to blood drawing. Finally we will review several cancer sites which offer a reasonable possibility of finding a major gene determining increased cancer susceptibility.

Methods of Linkage Analysis

The basic problem is to find the location of genes that determine susceptibility to the disease of interest. We attempt to find such genes by collecting information about pedigrees in which the disease appears to be segregating. This information includes the genetic relationships of the family members, indications of which family members are affected and other relevant clinical information. We also collect cells for DNA extraction so that we can examine inheritance; we use the term "marker" to denote a chromosome location which we can routinely assay to examine the inheritance from parents to offspring at that location. By definition, this location must be polymorphic and may be a gene but will usually be a chromosome region with no known coding function. We say that we have found "linkage" when one or more of these locations has been found to be close to a disease gene. Evidence of linkage comes from the observation of non-random segregation at a marker locus.

There are several statistical methodologies employed to identify linkage. First, the "classic" approach employs a segregation model which details the genetics of the disease-associated locus (Morton 1955; Ott 1988). This segregation model is obtained from observation of disease patterns within numerous families consisting minimally of those identified for the linkage study. Testing for linkage involves examining the recombination fraction, r, between the disease locus and a marker locus. The null hypothesis is free recombination between the loci (i.e. $r = 0.5$). Estimates of the recombination fraction numerically smaller than 0.5 and with sufficient statistical evidence generally imply that the marker and the disease locus are physically close.

The alternative approach is called the affected pair method (Penrose 1953; Suarez et al. 1978; Thomson 1986). The basis for considering the affected pair method is the HLA-association test where affected sibs are scored for their HLA concordance (share two alleles identical by descent (ibd), one allele ibd or zero alleles ibd). Under the null hypothesis of no association, the proportion of sibs in these categories should be 1/4, 1/2 and 1/4. Deviations imply non-random association and suggest linkage, although other interpretations are possible. The merit of the affected relative pair method is usually considered to be that the mode of inheritance prior to or during the analysis need not be understood. However, although the analysis does not require specification of the mode of inheritance, the power of the method is greatly dependent on this factor. Affected sib pair methods work well when the trait to be mapped is essentially recessive since information on two gametes is obtained from each pair (Bishop and Williamson 1990; Risch 1990b). However, when the trait is dominant, sib pair methods are less powerful since we expect the sib pairs to share one allele ibd under the null hypothesis. In this case, other relationships can be considerably more informative (Bishop and Williamson 1990; Risch 1990b). The most informative relationship, in general, for a dominant trait is the grandparent-grandchild relationship. Of course, in many practical situations this will not be a feasible design. Other more distant relationships can be more informative for linkage, but careful consideration of the number and type of markers to be typed needs to be made. For instance, cousins can be very informative for a candidate gene study, even for marker systems that are not highly polymorphic, but cousins are not particularly informative for a genomic search even for a highly polymorphic marker (Bishop and Williamson 1990; Risch 1990b).

The other limitation of this method relates to marker systems less polymorphic than HLA. As the HLA system is so informative, pairs of individuals are usually scored for their identity by descent concordance. For less polymorphic marker systems than the HLA system, even with parental information, only identity-by-state concordance can be scored, resulting in considerably less definitive information per pair of relatives (Lange 1986; Bishop and Williamson 1990). Therefore, the term "affected pair" should not be interpreted too literally. Other relatives can provide valuable information about the identity by descent status of the affected pair. Certainly, if there are other affected close relatives, these should be sampled. Also, though, unaffected relatives will add valuable information. For instance, consider two affected cousins who share an allele; if the allele is rare, then linkage is indicated, while if the allele is common, evidence for linkage will not be strong. Unfortunately, even if there is linkage, the second possibility is more likely than the first. However, sampling intervening relatives and confirming that they share the copy of that allele by descent rather than having two separate copies will make the linkage information as strong as if the shared allele were rare.

Problems of Linkage Analysis

What Is the Appropriate Phenotype for Linkage Analysis?

For linkage studies, we must minimally define a phenotype whose inheritance is consistent with a major gene. For rare diseases, we may not have much choice in either the phenotype or the pedigrees containing that phenotype. However, for more common diseases, there will be many pedigrees available and the difficulty arises in choosing the disease phenotype definition most indicative of a segregating disease-associated locus. In turn, we will use this definition to define the families most useful for linkage studies since we do not expect all pedigrees with few cases of the disease to be due to inherited susceptibility. Clues for such a major genetic effect must come from careful study of families. To perform these studies, we ascertain families by a proband, an individual with the cancer of interest, and look at the disease expression in relatives of this proband. While we expect the relatives to be at increased risk (with the higher risks obtained for closer genetic relationships), the pattern of increased risk by relationship determines both the feasibility of finding a major gene and the most likely mode of inheritance. Risch (1990a) has shown the specific algebraic formula between risks by degree of genetic relatedness for major gene inheritance. While we envisage that only rarely will sufficient family information be available to perform a formal goodness-of-fit test to these predictions, the latter are useful for eliminating gross deviations from further consideration.

More empirical evidence supporting genetic susceptibility may be derived from the identification of extended pedigrees where segregation through multiple generations and multiple branches within the pedigree can be observed. Such segregation is less likely to be due to environmental factors since distant cousinships will in general have few common environmental exposures.

Finally, examination of the pedigrees by clinical subtype or other tumour characteristics may suggest various etiologies, some of which are genetically determined. Such heterogeneity makes careful selection of pedigrees essential. A common feature for examination is the age at onset since many investigators have noted that inherited susceptibility produces earlier onset than the "common" form of the disease. The indication of the appropriateness of the phenotype should come from the observation of clearer patterns of inheritance within families than with the common form of the disease. This will usually be associated with an increased familial aggregation over the common form. For instance, with breast cancer where a rare, dominant gene for premenopausal disease is postulated, sisters of premenopausal cases have a higher risk of breast cancer than sisters of postmenopausal breast cancer cases.

The importance of a homogeneous subgroup can be evaluated by considering a simple model. Suppose we are considering a rare dominant disease which has two subforms, one of which is linked to a marker locus (and makes up a proportion p of families with this disease) while the other is unlinked. Numerical examination of this problem when the sampling unit is a nuclear family with four offspring and one affected parent shows that the average linkage information per family is a proportion p^2 of the information when there is only one form. Thus if 70% of the families are linked and 30% are unlinked, then the linkage information per family is one-half the information when all of the families are linked. Significant heterogeneity will preclude identification of linkage.

Premalignant Lesions and Preclinical Markers

One of the major problems of mapping disease loci is the age-specificity of the trait. Thus, individuals who are offspring of a recently affected individual are usually uninformative for linkage because they have not yet passed through the period of risk. As soon as they become affected or their age approaches the median age of onset of the cancer, then they will provide some linkage information; at present, their phenotype is essentially unknown. Preclinical markers and the presence of premalignant lesions offer an opportunity to score family members for their disease predisposition before the onset of the cancer. This has the advantage that, since the current generation will usually contain the largest number of individuals, a higher proportion of the population can be scored as being affected or unaffected with the disease. In addition, the information content of an individual pedigree can be greatly expanded. This approach has been particularly stressed by the Utah group (for instance, see Cannon-Albright et al., this volume). However, this approach does require the identification of an accurate preclinical marker. In the extreme case of adenomatous polyposis coli, an individual can usually be scored for the phenotype by their midteens. In more subtle cases, while individuals classified as affected but not carrying the disease gene will not seriously distort the analysis, if few in number, any significant number will destroy the possibility of finding linkage. In genetic terms, we are asking for a high genetic correlation between the cancer and the preclinical marker or presence of the precursor lesion.

The best-documented example of a preclinical marker is the adenomatous polyp for common colon cancer. Detailed studies of family history of colorectal cancer among relatives of colorectal cancer cases as compared to the family history of colorectal cancer among the relatives of individuals with adenomas have shown essentially similar results, namely a relative risk of approximately 2.3 as compared to the family members of probands without disease (Bishop and Burt 1990). This shows that the adenoma and a colorectal cancer have the same impact on the risk of disease in the relatives and, for the purposes of linkage analysis, can be considered as the same trait; that is, both individuals with an adenoma and individuals with colorectal cancer can be considered to be affected for the purposes of linkage analysis.

Presence of Related Phenotypes Within the Pedigrees

A related problem to the discussion of preclinical phenotypes is the presence of other phenotypes within the pedigrees. For instance, in breast cancer families collected for multiple cases of premenopausal cancer, there will invariably be cases of postmenopausal cancer. Claus (1989) has shown that, at least among first degree relatives of premenopausal probands, there is a high genetic correlation between both forms of breast cancer suggesting that the two cases have the same genetic etiology. Schildkraut et al. (1989) have also shown a high genetic correlation between ovarian cancer and breast cancer but found no evidence of a correlation between endometrial cancer and either ovarian or breast cancer. Again, decisions of the appropriate definitions of phenotype require extensive analysis of families prior to linkage analysis in specific families.

Extended Pedigrees or Affected Pairs of Relatives: Which is the Appropriate Sampling Unit?

The next issue to confront an investigator preparing a gene-mapping study is the structure of the families to be studied. Discussions are often centred on the advantages of extended pedigrees compared to affected pairs of relatives although too much attention is usually focused on the method of analysis rather than the optimal study unit. An informed discussion of the choice of sampling unit requires knowledge of the mode of inheritance of the disease. Several specific aspects of the mode of inheritance are important. First, the decision as to whether the trait appears to be recessive or dominant. This can be addressed by comparing the risk to a sibling of a proband with the parent of the proband. If the two risks are comparable (and, of course, greater than the population risk) then this would suggest that an underlying major gene is dominant while a sibling risk much greater than the parental risk would imply recessive inheritance of a major gene.

For recessive traits, many of the families ascertained will consist of only sibships. For these, sampling of the relevant nuclear families (including the parents) is all that is required. The exception to this is when there is inbreeding, as would be the case for a rare recessive disease in which case individuals within the inbreeding loop should also be sampled whenever possible.

For a dominant trait, the frequency of the trait and the expression of the postulated gene will determine the size of the relevant sampling unit. Strictly, the important feature of the mode of inheritance is the allele frequency rather than the frequency of the trait. For traits with a high allele frequency, families whose only affected members have distant relationships are unlikely to share a common genetic etiology and so are not useful for linkage analysis. Sampling units should then involve closer relationships, such as uncle-nephew or grandparent-grand-child relationships. These units can be tied together to form an extended pedigree. Alternatively, if segregation can be followed through many branches of a large pedigree then there is a considerable pay-off in statistical terms in favour of extensive sampling of this pedigree. The merit of the extended pedigree approach is that if there are different genetic loci underlying the susceptibility then large families with many affected individuals are more likely to elucidate etiology than many small families.

Second, we need to be concerned about the genetic homogeneity of the trait. Of particular relevance is the variation in phenotype within pedigrees as com-pared to between pedigrees. If there is evidence of phenotypic heterogeneity between pedigrees then we should direct attention towards sampling particular subtypes with a view to examining linkage in the other subtypes when a candidate locus for linkage has been identified. This approach is appropriate especially when one subtype is rare compared with the other, since a candidate study requires only six informative meioses to confirm linkage at a significance level of 0.05. Using this approach, effort is made to map the common form while confirming the linkage with the rarer form.

Logistical Problems

Linkage analysis of diseases suffers from numerous logistical problems. We will review each of these in turn and consider methods that partially solve them.

Availability of Pedigrees

This is the most serious constraint; if there are only a small number of pedigrees available, there is no linkage study. The reasons why pedigrees may be un-available include rareness of the disease, prereproductive mortality or lack of familial aggregation. Even if there is increased familial aggregation, there should be some indication of mendelian inheritance after allowing for partial penetrance before a linkage study can be justified.

Availability of Pedigrees but Unavailability of Individuals

Linkage analysis takes most of its information from examination of vertical transmission and especially evidence of transmission between affected in-dividuals. Demographic constraints usually restrict the number of generations currently alive in the general population to three but the age-dependent nature of cancer expression will normally restrict the number of generations of affected individuals to two. Additional information on a pedigree will then be required since a pedigree consisting of only a parent-offspring pair is uninformative for linkage.

Next, increased mortality due to the disease under study will have further impact on the availability of individuals for sampling. For studies of families expressing solid tumours, there is some hope because of the development of the polymerase chain reaction (PCR) technique and its application to stored specimens, especially paraffin block material. Pathologists have been storing tumours fixed in paraffin blocks since the end of the last century and these blocks represent a valuable source of material for genotyping an individual. The PCR technique allows the chemical replication of DNA, even in partially degraded form, to allow marker typing. The technique requires at least partial sequence knowledge for the marker and the production of synthetic oligonucleotides to match key elements of the sequence. While this information is rarely available for current markers, many investigators are beginning to routinely sequence their probes because of the economics and efficiency of PCR technology even when ample material is available (for instance, Kidd et al. 1989). For linkage analysis, this technique will be useful for adding information to preliminary results which show a possibility of linkage. The limited amount of DNA available from paraffin blocks will not allow random genomic searches from these samples. Finally, for this approach, the major problem can become one of resources needed to track down the blocks. In the United Kingdom, many hospitals keep blocks for limited periods and, as there is no central registry of these samples, effort is required to track down the institution holding the samples or the location of the samples even when the institution is known.

Finally, other factors may restrict the informativeness of the pedigrees. Divorce, non-paternity, unwillingness to provide blood samples and early mortality through factors independent of the disease are all routinely encountered. This means that if a relative is alive and agrees to participate and the family is particularly informative, the investigator must be willing to go to extreme lengths to get the sample. In the Imperial Cancer Research Fund Genetic Epidemiology Laboratory based in Leeds, during a six-month period, we have obtained samples from Barcelona, Buenos Aires, California, Northern Canada, Colorado, various parts of France, Ireland and Kathmandu. The possibility of mapping is also greatly improved by the availability of large families and a stable population; this is one of the major reasons for the success of the studies conducted in Utah (Cannon-Albright et al., this volume).

Methods of Statistical Analysis

There are important decisions to be made before or during a linkage analysis with regard to phenotype. As linkage analysis requires the specification of a disease phenotype (affected, unaffected or unknown) and the analysis may be quite sensitive to these assumptions, careful consideration is necessary. Essentially the solution depends upon the appropriateness of the linkage model to the situation being investigated. In particular, the assumption of levels of phenocopies (cases of the cancer not due to genetic factors) has a major bearing on the lod scores. For instance, if we assume that there are no phenocopies then any phenocopy will be interpreted as a recombination event in the analysis. If there are too many recombinations, then all evidence for linkage is destroyed. On the other hand, assuming too high a level of phenocopies will produce numerically smaller lod scores than appropriate and make successful mapping more difficult.

Another problem encountered is the specification of the mode of inheritance. While, on average, the true statistical model will best reflect the evidence for linkage, there is now reasonable empirical evidence (Risch et al. 1990) and limited theoretical arguments (Clerget-Darpoux et al. 1986) for believing that a broad range of genetic models give similar linkage results. While all of these terms lack precision such that definitive statements are not possible, the most important feature of the genetic model appears to be the level of dominance assumed. That is, analysing a dominant trait as a recessive or vice versa can eliminate any evidence of linkage, while misspecifying the degree of penetrance for a dominant trait will not substantially affect the linkage results (Clerget-Darpoux et al. 1986). Currently, most investigators analyse a complex trait as a partially penetrant dominant as well as a partially penetrant recessive trait allowing for reasonable levels of penetrance. However, we should note that considering a variety of models requires suitable statistical allowance since the lod score limit of 3.0 to conclude linkage assumes optimization only over the recombination fraction. The limit must be increased above 3.0 if optimization occurs over both penetrance and recombination.

For modes of inheritance without phenocopies, an additional approach is to analyse the disease with extremely low penetrance (e.g. 10%). This has the effect of measuring the linkage information available from examination of the affected individuals eliminating linkage information from unaffected individuals. Comparison between the lod scores for linkage and the estimates of recombination fraction for the complete model and the model with severely reduced penetrance gives an indication of the basis of the linkage information obtained from the pedigree. If the evidence is similar then the linkage information is coming mainly from the affected individuals since unaffected individuals will be essentially uninformative when low penetrance is assumed. Large discrepancies indicate that linkage information is being obtained from the unaffected individuals.

Studies of Specific Sites

Breast Cancer

Particular attention is being focused on breast cancer at present with many laboratories collecting families for linkage studies. For many years, the familial aggregation of breast cancer and especially premenopausal breast cancer has been noted. While the risk to a female first degree relative of a breast cancer case ranges from 1.5 to 3.0 depending upon the onset age of the case, the risks to a relative of two first degree breast cancer cases is 8.5 (Claus 1989). This is consistent with and suggestive of a rare dominant major gene segregating within these families (Risch, personal communication). This is also supported by analysis of extended pedigrees found in the clinical setting which could also be examples of pedigrees segregating a dominant gene (e.g. Williams and Anderson 1984; Bishop et al. 1988). Statistical support within a single pedigree for this assertion is rarely obtained since sex-specific penetrance and late age of onset cloud the issue of mode of inheritance.

The difficulties of linkage analysis within these pedigrees has been discussed in other parts of this manuscript.

Colon Cancer

Considerable interest is also being focused on colon cancer. Bodmer et al. (1987) mapped the gene responsible for adenomatous polyposis coli (APC) to 5q. While APC is comparatively rare, the same gene has been shown to be important in the carcinogenesis events for common colorectal cancer with over 60% of all cancers showing a deletion of the APC gene (Ashton-Rickardt et al. 1989). Another locus deleted in many colorectal cancers and located on chromosome 18 is close to the Kidd blood group for which Lynch et al. (1985) found interesting but not confirmatory evidence of linkage for cancer family syndrome. Leppert et al. (1990) have also identified a family which apparently segregates a form of site-specific colon cancer which mapped to the APC locus. Further examination of this pedigree suggests a form of APC with highly variable numbers of polyps since several members of the family would be clinically considered to have APC. The linkage mapping of colon cancer is therefore aimed at specific sites, the APC locus, the chromosome 18 gene and the region of chromosome 17 containing the p53 tumour protein, a site of frequent deletion and mutation of colorectal tumours. Mecklin (1987) has estimated that 5% of colorectal cancers are inherited as autosomal dominants. The contribution of each of the above loci to this total is not yet known.

Ovarian Cancer

Analysis of the Utah Genealogical Database has shown that ovarian cancer is the third most familial of all the common cancers (Cannon et al. 1982), exceeding both colon cancer and breast cancer in familial aggregation. Schildkraut et al. (1989) found a relative risk of nearly three for ovarian cancer in the first degree relatives of ovarian cancer probands. In practice, while ovarian cancer families are rare, the families are often impressive in terms of the number of cases represented in the pedigree and the number of generations over which these pedigrees extend. An autosomal dominant mode of inheritance is compatible with the family patterns. Unfortunately, the high mortality from ovarian cancer greatly reduces the availability of readily informative families.

There are also families segregating both ovarian and breast cancer. Schildkraut et al. (1989) found a high genetic correlation between these two sites confirming the observations of various clinical investigators (for instance, Go et al. 1983). Families segregating both breast and ovarian cancer should therefore also be considered as candidates for linkage studies.

Discussion

The success achieved in mapping the rarer mendelian diseases has encouraged the initiation of many linkage studies with the optimistic view that by localizing an important gene for a disease we will be able to approach disease etiology by examining the product of that gene. A mutated or absent product may suggest screening schemes for the disease or even therapies. Although the molecular approach is becoming clearer, there are a number of difficulties that face the genetic epidemiologist. Primarily, the problem is this: How to define or find a trait that is determined by a major gene. Success in this ensures that there is some prospect of finding that gene although other confounding problems, such as genetic heterogeneity or lack of pedigrees, may negate that prospect. Failure to identify a mendelian trait will result in no prospect of ever finding a gene although spurious results may suggest linkage. Subsequent lack of replication will follow, to everyone's frustration.

The only way to produce such a trait is by careful examination of pedigrees prior to linkage analysis. There are many levels at which we have to discuss this problem. First, we should examine many families to identify the possibility of mendelian inheritance and, if found, the most likely mode of inheritance. The risks to relatives of probands give us an adequate measure for deciding upon the mode of inheritance. Second, some subforms may show differing patterns of familial aggregation. Standard factors to examine are age and laterality for paired organs under the assumption that genetically predisposed individuals are expected to express earlier and more completely than sporadic forms. Finally, if the families are still not adequate for linkage analysis, we can search for predisposing lesions, preclinical markers or alternative expression of the putative gene in terms of other cancer sites that may make the families more informative. Confirmation of a high genetic correlation between the site of interest and the related phenotypes is required to permit a joint definition of the affected phenotype.

Other issues related to mapping have not been discussed but should be noted. Primarily these involve the method of analysis which should require making a definition of phenotype prior to marker analysis and awareness of the statistical costs involved in computing linkage results over a variety of genetic models. Either of these aspects is liable to produce false-positive results. Although we have concentrated on affected pair methods and classic linkage, analytical methods involving model-free assumptions for extended pedigrees have been developed (Weeks and Lange 1989).

Finally, we should note that analysis of complex diseases will involve large-scale collaborative efforts since adequate families, even for common cancers, will rarely be available to a single investigator. Excessive disease-associated mortality and the geographical spread of family members make such collaborations necessary to provide sufficient family material.

Acknowledgments. The authors would like to thank Drs. Neil Risch and Doug Easton for many discussions related to this and related subjects and also to Sir Walter Bodmer for comments on this manuscript.

References

Ashton-Rickardt PG, Dunlop MG, Nakamura Y, Morris RG, Purdie CA, Steel CM, Evans HJ, Bird CC, Wyllie AH (1989) High frequency of APC loss in sporadic colorectal carcinoma due to breaks clustered in 5q21–q22. Oncogene 4:1169–1174

Barker DF, Wright E, Nguyen K, Cannon L, Fain P, Goldgar D, Bishop DT, Carey J, Baty B, Kivlin J, Willard H, Waye JS, Greig G, Leinwand L, Nakamura Y, O'Connell P, Leppert M, Lalouel J-M, White R, Skolnick M (1987) The gene for NF1 (von Recklinghausen neurofibromatosis) is in the pericentromeric region of chromosome 17. Science 236:1100–1102

Bishop DT, Burt RW (1990) Genetic epidemiology and molecular genetics of colorectal adenomas and cancer. In: Rozen P (ed) Frontiers of gastrointestinal research. Karger, Basel

Bishop DT, Williamson JA (1990) The power of identity-by-state methods for linkage analysis. Am J Hum Genet 46:254–265

Bishop DT, Cannon-Albright L, McLellan T, Gardner EJ, Skolnick MH (1988) Segregation and linkage analysis of nine Utah breast cancer pedigrees. Genet Epidemiol 5:151–169

Bodmer WF (1990) Hereditary colorectal cancer – a commentary. In: Proceedings of Fourth International Symposium on Colorectal Cancer, Kobe, Japan, November 1989. Springer, Tokyo

Bodmer WF, Bailey CJ, Bodner J, Bussey HJR, Ellis A, Gorman P, Lucibello FC, Murday VA, Rider SH, Scambler P, Sheer D, Solomon E, Spurr NK (1987) Localization of the gene for familial adenomatous polyposis on chromosome 5. Nature 328:614–616

Botstein D, White RL, Skolnick M, Davis RW (1980) Construction of a genetic linkage map in man using restriction fragment length polymorphisms. Am J Hum Genet 32:314–331

Cannon L, Bishop DT, Skolnick M, Hunt S, Lyon JL, Smart CR (1982) Genetic epidemiology of prostate cancer in the Utah Mormon Genealogy. Cancer Surveys 1:47–69

Claus E (1989) Age of onset and the inheritance of breast cancer. PhD dissertation, Yale University

Clerget-Darpoux F, Bonaïti-Pellie C, Hochez J (1986) Effects of misspecifying genetic parameters in lod score analysis. Biometrics 42:393–400

Go RCP, King MC, Bailey-Wilson J, Elston RC, Lynch HT (1983) Genetic epidemiology of breast cancer and associated cancers in high risk pedigrees. I. Segregation analysis. J Natl Cancer Inst 71:455–461

Gusella JF, Wexler NS, Commeally PM, Naylor SL, Anderson MA, Tanzi RE, Watkins PC, Ottina K, Wallace MR, Sakaguchi AY, Young AB, Shoulson I, Bonilla E, Martin JB (1983) A polymorphic DNA marker genetically linked to Huntington's Disease. Nature 306:234–238

Kidd KK, Bowcock AW, Schmidtke J, Track RK, Ricciuti F, Hutchings G, Bale A, Pearson P, Willard HF (1989) Report of the DNA committee and catalogs of clones and mapped genes and DNA polymorphisms. Human Gene Mapping 10: Tenth International Workshop on Human Gene Mapping. Cytogenet Cell Genet 51:622–947

Lange K (1986) The affected sib pair method using identity by state relations. Am J Hum Genet 39:148–150

Leppert M, Burt R, Hughes JP, Samowitz W, Nakamura Y, Woodward S, Gardner EJ, Lalouel J-M, White R (1990) Genetic analysis of an inherited predisposition to colon cancer in a family with an inherited number of adenomatous polyps. N Engl J Med 322:904–908

Lynch HT, Schuelke GS, Kimberling WJ, Albano WA, Lynch JF, Biscone KA, Lipkin ML, Deschner EE, Mikol YB, Sandberg AA, Elston RC, Bailey-Wilson JE, Danes BS (1985) Hereditary non-polyposis colorectal cancer (Lynch syndromes I and II): II. Biomarker studies. Cancer 56:939–951

Mecklin JP (1987) Frequency of hereditary colorectal carcinoma. Gastroenterol 93:1021–1025

Morton NE (1955) Sequential tests for the detection of linkage. Am J Hum Genet 7:277–318

Ott J (1988) Analysis of human genetic linkage. Johns Hopkins University Press, Baltimore

Penrose LS (1953) The general purpose sib-pair linkage test. Ann Eugenics 6:133–138

Risch N (1990a) Linkage strategies for genetically complex traits. I. Multilocus models. Am J Hum Genet 46:222–228

Risch N (1990b) Linkage strategies for genetically complex traits. II. The power of affected relative pairs. Am J Hum Genet 46:229–241

Risch N, Claus E, Giuffra L (1990) Genetic Analysis Workshop VI: analysis of simulations. Gen Epidemiol

Schildkraut JM, Risch N, Thompson WD (1989) Evaluating genetic association among ovarian, breast, and endometrial cancer: evidence for a breast/ovarian cancer relationship. Am J Hum Genet 45:521–529

Solomon E, Bodmer WF (1979) Evolution of sickle variant gene. Lancet 923

Solomon E, Voss R, Hall V, Bodmer WF, Jass JR, Jeffreys AJ, Lucibello FC, Patel I, Rider SH (1987) Chromosome 5 allele loss in human colorectal carcinomas. Nature 328:616–619

Suarez BK, Rice J, Reich T (1978) The generalized sib pair IBD distributions: its use in the detection of linkage. Ann Hum Genet 42:87–94

Thomson G (1986) Determining the mode of inheritance of RFLP-associated diseases using the affected sib-pair. Am J Hum Genet 42:315–326

Tsui L-C, Buchwald M, Barker D, Braman JC, Knowlton R, Schumm JW, Eiberg H, Mohr J, Kennedy D, Plavsic N, Zsiga M, Markiewicz D, Akots G, Brown V, Helms C, Gravius T, Parker C, Rediker K, Donis-Keller H (1985) Cystic fibrosis locus defined by a genetically linked DNA marker. Science 230:1054–1057

Weeks DE, Lange K (1989) The affected-pedigree-member method of linkage analysis. Am J Hum Genet 42:315–326

Williams WR, Anderson DE (1984) Genetic epidemiology of breast cancer segregation analysis of 200 Danish pedigrees. Genet Epidemiol 1:7–20

Genetic Epidemiology of Retinoblastoma

C. Bonaïti-Pellié, F. Clerget-Darpoux, and M.-C. Babron

Introduction

The retinoblastoma story provides a very good example of a case where mechanisms assessed by genetic epidemiology were confirmed several years later by molecular genetics. There are still some questions raised by the analysis of family data which remain unsolved and for which molecular genetic approaches will probably provide the expected answers.

Retinoblastoma is a malignant embryonal tumor of the eye that affects approximately one in 20 000 children, most often before the age of 4 years. Familial aggregation has been reported for a long time; several comprehensive surveys were conducted in the period 1950–1970, leading to the conclusion that there are two types of retinoblastoma, hereditary and non-hereditary (sporadic). A good review can be found in Vogel (1979).

The Two-Mutation Hypothesis

The sporadic type of retinoblastoma is always unilateral whereas the hereditary type is more often bilateral and is dominantly inherited with a high degree of penetrance. All bilateral cases and only some unilateral cases are thus carriers of a gene which was transmitted from a carrier (affected or not) parent or was the result of a new mutation. A unifying model was proposed by Knudson (1971) who hypothesized that only two mutational events were necessary for tumor formation, the first of which can be germinal (in the hereditary type) or somatic in retinal cells (in the sporadic type). When the first mutation is germinal, all the cells, in particular the retinal cells, carry the mutation. The second event would always be somatic and would lead to tumor formation in each cell having acquired the two successive mutations. The occurrence of two somatic mutations in the same retinal cell is a very rare event and even rarer in both eyes. Thus sporadic cases are never bilateral. Knudson tested his hypothesis using two kinds of data. First he found that the proportion of bilaterally, unilaterally, and unaffected individuals among gene carriers was in accord with each tumor resulting from a single somatic

Unité de recherches d'épidémiologie génétique (U. 155 INSERM), Château du Longchamp, Bois de Boulogne, 75016 Paris, France

H.T. Lynch and P. Tautu (Eds.)
Recent Progress
in the Genetic Epidemiology of Cancer
© Springer-Verlag Berlin Heidelberg 1991

event that occurs in a stochastic fashion. Indeed, in such a case, the number of tumors should follow a Poisson distribution. Comparing the proportions of bilaterally, unilaterally, and unaffected individuals among gene carriers, with the proportions inferred from the expected distribution of tumors for various Poisson means, he found a fairly good fit for a mean number of tumors equal to three. Second, he analyzed the ages at diagnosis for the two forms of retinoblastoma and showed that the proportion of cases not yet diagnosed at various ages declined in accord with a "one-hit" curve in bilateral cases, and with a "two-hit" curve in isolated unilateral cases.

Molecular genetic approaches supported this hypothesis and enabled the precise determination of the locus involved in the disease.

The Retinoblastoma Gene

On the basis that a few patients carried a small constitutional deletion on chromosome 13 (13q14), a mutation at a locus in this region was suspected to be the first event. This was demonstrated by Sparkes et al. (1983) who found tight linkage between retinoblastoma and esterase D, the locus of which maps also on 13q14. This locus was called the Rb1 locus.

The nature of the second event was examined by using esterase D polymorphisms (Godbout et al. 1983) and restriction fragment length polymorphisms (RFLPs) located on chromosome 13 (Cavenee et al. 1983; Dryja et al. 1984). Comparing genotypes in the patients' lymphocytes and in their tumor led to the assessment that the second event was a functional loss of the homologous normal allele at the Rb1 locus in a retinal cell. It appeared that the tumor was the result of complete loss of normal gene at this locus and that the mutant allele behaved recessively at the cellular level. This was the first evidence for a tumor suppressor gene, which was called an antioncogene in contrast to the oncogene with its activator role (Knudson 1983). A few years later, the gene was isolated and characterized by three groups of workers (Friend et al. 1986; Fung et al. 1987; Lee et al. 1987).

Parental Origin of the Germinal Mutation

The difference in the germ cell development of males and females can induce a sex difference in mutation rates. All female gametes can be formed by as few as 23 cell divisions occurring before birth, whereas in males several hundred cell divisions are needed (Vogel and Rathenberg 1975). If germinal mutation occurs in connection with DNA replication, a higher mutation rate in males than in females can be predicted. Since mutant genes would accumulate in the stem cell pool with time, a linear increase of mutation rate with paternal age is expected. Seventeen years ago, we used this property to investigate whether bilateral isolated cases could be due to germinal mutations resulting from a gene-copying error (Pellié et al. 1973). We found an increased paternal age (and no effect of maternal age) in bilateral isolated cases and not in unilateral cases, suggesting that the isolated bilateral form was caused by a new germinal mutation with a higher mutation rate in males than in females.

This result was recently confirmed by Dryja et al. (1989) and Zhu et al. (1989) using molecular biology techniques to identify the parental origin of the mutation in respectively ten and five patients with isolated bilateral retinoblastoma. Among these 15 de novo mutations, 14 (respectively 10 and 4) were found to occur on the paternal chromosome 13, showing a significant excess of paternal compared with maternal origin of new mutations ($p = 0.001$).

The same excess of paternal origin of fresh germinal mutations was found in microscopically detectable deletions by Ejima et al. (1988): in eight of the nine informative cases, the abnormal chromosome was derived from the father ($p = 0.04$).

Penetrance and Expressivity

The existence of families with distant relatives affected by retinoblastoma was first pointed out by Neel (1962). These cases with at least two unaffected carriers represent more than one-fourth of all families with several affected individuals in our series (Briard-Guillemot et al. 1974). This is poorly compatible with the quasi-complete penetrance inferred from the study of the offspring of bilateral cases, which implies that a gene carrier would have a very small probability of somatic mutation never occurring in any of his retinal cells. Neel (1962) suggested that these families could be exhibiting the phenomenon of delayed mutation, a hypothesis which was originally proposed by Auerbach (1956) for explaining familial observations in a type of split-hand. A premutated allele could be transmitted through one or several generations and then changed into a mutated allele [what Hermann (1977) calls telomutation] either in the retinal cells of a subject who could then have retinoblastoma, or in a germ cell producing an affected offspring.

On the other hand, Ellsworth (1969) and Matsunaga (1976) suggested that the risk for the offspring could be different according to the expressivity in the carrier parent: the offspring of individuals exhibiting the most severe form of the disease (bilateral cases) would have a higher risk of being affected (higher penetrance) and more chance of having a bilateral form if they are affected (higher degree of expressivity) than the offspring of individuals with a less severe form (unilateral cases). The offspring of unaffected carriers, who have the smallest degree of expressivity, would have the smallest penetrance and expressivity. Hermann (1976, 1977) postulated that the phenomenon of delayed mutation could entirely explain these differences. According to Matsunaga (1978), such differences would be due to different degrees of "host resistance" among gene carriers: an individual carrying the retinoblastoma gene would be more or less susceptible to tumor development, and the occurrence of a second mutation would be unnecessary. This susceptibility would be partly genetically determined with polygenic inheritance and two thresholds subdividing the population of gene carriers into three possible phenotypes: unaffected, unilaterally, and bilaterally affected.

We investigated these hypotheses (Bonaïti-Pellié and Briard-Guillemot 1981) using 166 pedigrees belonging to nine series of the literature, including our own series (Falls and Neel 1951; Tucker et al. 1957; Vogel 1957; Macklin 1960; Schappert-Kimmijser et al. 1966; Ellsworth 1969; Sorsby 1972; Briard-Guillemot et al. 1974; Matsunaga and Ogyu 1976).

In a first step, we could confirm the higher risk for offspring when the gene carrier parent was bilaterally affected (0.49) than unilaterally or unaffected (0.24), as well as a higher proportion of bilateral cases among affected offsping of bilateral parents (0.87) than unilateral (0.76) and unaffected carrier parents (0.60). In addition, even having carefully taken into account the ascertainment mode of families, we found that the offspring of unaffected and unilateral carriers were at significantly higher risk when they already had an affected sib.

In a second step, we assumed two types of transmitters among unilateral and unaffected gene carriers — low transmitters (presumably bearing a premutation) and high transmitters (bearing the complete mutation). We found that, among high transmitters, there still remained a different risk for the offspring of bilaterally affected individuals on the one hand (0.49) and unilaterally and unaffected individuals on the other hand (0.31), which argued against the hypothesis that delayed mutation can entirely explain the differences in penetrance and expressivity.

The Balanced Insertion Hypothesis

A possible explanation of the instances of familial transmission of retinoblastoma through healthy parents was provided by cytogenetic studies. Riccardi et al. (1979), Rivera et al. (1981), Strong et al. (1981), and Turleau et al. (1983) reported cases of balanced insertion which give rise in the offspring to either a 13q14-trisomy, or a 13q14-deletion with retinoblastoma, or a balanced insertion. This could provide a cytogenetic explanation for the delayed mutation hypothesis, the balanced insertion representing the premutation and the 13q14 monosomy the complete mutation. Using the same series of the literature, we reanalyzed the data to test the hypothesis that this mechanism could explain all the differences in disease segregation among families (Bonaïti-Pellié et al. 1991).

The probabilities for families have been computed assuming three genotypes: the carriers of the balanced inserton (B carriers), the carriers of the deletion (D carriers), and the normal genotype (including the 13q14 trisomics who are known to have a normal phenotype). Three possible phenotypes were considered: unaffected, unilaterally, and bilaterally affected individuals. We assumed that all bilateral cases are D carriers and we neglected the occurrence of sporadic cases in the families.

To test if the differences of disease segregation among families can be entirely explained by balanced insertions, we performed homogeneity tests according to the phenotype of the carrier parent in nuclear families under the two different hypotheses: (1) equal viability of gametes, and (2) smaller viability of unbalanced gametes.

Assuming equal viability of gametes, we found a significant heterogeneity among families according to the phenotype of the carrier parent ($X_4^2 = 13.61, p < 0.01$), with no difference between unilateral and unaffected parents. Allowing for smaller viability of unbalanced gametes led to a similar difference among families and homogeneity was significantly rejected ($X_8^2 = 20.26, p < 0.02$). We noted also that, under the hypothesis of balanced insertion, equal viability of gametes could be strongly rejected ($X_2^2 = 22.27, p \ll 0.001$).

Thus, this analysis showed that balanced chromosomal insertion of the 13q14 region cannot entirely explain the differences in penetrance and expressivity observed in the offspring of gene carriers according to their phenotypes.

Other Hypotheses

Balanced insertion of the 13q14 region has been shown to account for some instances of transmission of retinoblastoma through healthy parents. However, familial segregation of the disease cannot be explained by this phenomenon alone. This is probably a rare event, and other mechanisms must be involved.

First, the probability of the second event and consequently of tumor formation for a gene carrier could be genetically determined depending on other loci than the Rb 1 mutation. This hypothesis presents some similarities with the host resistance theory of Matsunaga (1978) who argued, however, that there was little need to postulate a second event. We indirectly investigated this hypothesis by studying the proportion of cancer deaths in grandparents of patients with retinoblastoma (Bonaïti-Pellié and Briard-Guillemot 1980). We found an excess of cancer deaths, suggesting the existence of a non-specific factor of susceptibility to cancer. However, studying this excess in the paternal and the maternal sides of family patients on the one hand, and in different pedigree patterns on the other hand, we found arguments for this factor acting on the first mutation, and not influencing the mutation rate of the second event in gene carriers.

Second, the probability of tumor formation could depend on the nature of the germinal mutation D. Suppose that mutation Di induces a greater probability of somatic recombination or of abnormal chromosomal segregation at mitosis than mutation Dj, then the probability of tumor formation will be greater for Di than for Dj carriers. One may also postulate with Knudson (1983) that the second event could lead to a cell with smaller viability when occurring in a Dj than in a Di carrier: if an allele lethal at the cellular level was present at some other locus on the chromosome 13 homologue, occurrence of a deletion including this locus at the other chromosome 13 copy would lead to cell death, and no tumor would result. Dryja et al. (1984) suggested a similar explanation for the observation made by Matsunaga (1980) that the incidence of bilateral retinoblastoma was lower in patients with a constitutional microscopically detectable 13q14 deletion than that in non-deletion patients.

In the first hypothesis, the probability of tumor formation in a gene carrier would depend on the genotype of both parents, and therefore would vary from one generation to another. In the second hypothesis, whatever the mechanisms involved in the probability of tumor formation (different probabilities of the second event, or smaller viability of some cells having acquired this second event), this probability would remain unchanged from one generation of gene carrier to the next one. The data available at the present time permit no discrimination between these two hypotheses, since testing the equality of probability of tumor formation for successive generations in the same family is not possible.

Molecular biology could help to investigate such hypotheses. As far as we are aware, there is only one study where unaffected gene carriers were detected through the analysis of DNA markers both within and flanking the Rb gene on chromosome 13 (Scheffer et al. 1989). Among 19 families with hereditary retinoblastoma, there were 18 informative families. In two of them, an unaffected gene carrier was evidenced in the last generation. In none of these families was the nature of the mutation identified, except for one other family where three individuals exhibited a deletion of the whole gene, all of them being affected.

Thus, so far, there is no argument from molecular genetics for discriminating between the above hypotheses. One method of investigation would be to study two kinds of pedigrees strongly selected on the existence of either several unaffected carriers with mostly unilateral involvement on the one hand, or on a regular transmission of the disease with mostly bilateral involvement on the other hand. Systematic studies of the nature of the inherited mutation in these two kinds of pedigrees would probably provide the answer to this important question. It would also permit the detection of possible balanced insertions at the molecular level (not detectable on karyotype) and evaluation of the relative frequency of this mechanism.

References

Auerbach C (1956) A possible case of delayed mutation in man. Ann Hum Genet 20:266–269
Bonaiti-Pellié C, Briard-Guillemot ML (1980) Excess of cancer deaths in grandparents of patients with retinoblastoma. J Med Genet 17:95–101
Bonaiti-Pellié C, Briard-Guillemot ML (1981) Segregation analysis in hereditary retinoblastoma. Hum Genet 57:411–419
Bonaiti-Pellié C, Clerget-Darpoux F, Babron MC (1991) Hereditary retinoblastoma: can balanced insertion entirely explain the differences of expressivity among families? Hum Genet (in press)
Briard-Guillemot ML, Bonaiti-Pellié C, Feingold J, Frézal J (1974) Etude génétique du rétinoblastome. Hum Genet 24:271–284
Cavenee WK, Dryja TP, Phillips RA, Benedict WF, Godbout R, Gallie BL, Murphree AL, Strong LC, White RL (1983) Expression of recessive alleles by chromosomal mechanisms in retinoblastoma. Nature 305:779–784
Dryja TP, Cavenee W, White R, Rapaport JM, Peterson R, Albert DM, Bruns GAP (1984)

Homozygosity of chromosome 13 in retinoblastoma. N Engl J Med 310:550–553

Dryja TP, Mukai S, Petersen R, Rapaport JM, Walton D, Yandell DW (1989) Parental origin of mutations of the retinoblastoma gene. Nature 339:556–558

Ejima Y, Sasaki MS, Kaneko A, Tanooka H (1988) Types, rates, origin and expressivity of mutations involving 13q14 in retinoblastoma patients. Hum Genet 79:118–123

Ellsworth RM (1969) The practical management of retinoblastoma. Trans Am Ophthalmol Soc 67:462–534

Falls HF, Neel JV (1951) Genetics of retinoblastoma. Arch Ophthalmol 46:367–389

Friend SH, Bernards R, Rogelji S, Weinberg RA, Rapaport JM, Albert DM, Dryja TP (1986) A human DNA segment with properties of the gene that predisposes to retinoblastoma and osteosarcoma. Nature 323:643–646

Fung YKT, Murphree AL, T'Ang A, Qian J, Hinrichs SH, Benedict WF (1987) Structural evidence for the authenticity of the human retinoblastoma gene. Science 236:1657–1661

Godbout R, Dryja TP, Squirre J, Gallie BL, Phillips RA (1983) Somatic inactivation of genes on chromosome 13 is a common event in retinoblastoma. Nature 304:451–453

Hermann J (1976) Delayed mutation as a cause of retinoblastoma: application to genetic counseling. Birth Defects 12:79–90

Hermann J (1977) Delayed mutation model: Carotid body tumors and retinoblastoma. In: Mulvihill JJ, Miller RW, Fraumeni JF (eds) Genetics of human cancer. Raven, New York, p 417

Knudson AG (1971) Mutation and cancer: statistical study of retinoblastoma. Proc Natl Acad Sci USA 68:820–823

Knudson AG (1983) Model hereditary cancers of man. Prog Nucleic Acid Res Mol Biol 29:17–25

Lee WH, Bookstein R, Hong F, Young LH, Shew JY, Lee EYHP (1987) Human retinoblastoma susceptibility gene: cloning, identification and sequence. Science 235:1394–1399

Macklin MT (1960) A study of retinoblastoma in Ohio. Am J Hum Genet 12:1–43

Matsunaga E (1976) Hereditary retinoblastoma: penetrance, expressivity and age at onset. Hum Genet 33:1–15

Matsunaga E (1978) Hereditary retinoblastoma: delayed mutation or host resistance? Am J Hum Genet 30:406–424

Matsunaga E (1980) Retinoblastoma: host resistance and 13q-chromosomal deletion. Hum Genet 56:53–58

Matsunaga E, Ogyu H (1976) Retinoblastoma in Japan: follow up survey of sporadic cases. Jpn J Ophthalmol 20:266–282

Neel JV (1962) Mutations in the human population. In: Burdette WJ (ed) Methodology in human genetics. Holden Day, San Francisco, p 203

Pellié C, Briard ML, Feingold J, Frézal J (1973) Parental age in retinoblastoma. Hum Genet 20:59–62

Riccardi VM, Hittner HM, Francke U, Pippin S, Holmquist GP, Kretzer FL, Ferrell R (1979) Partial triplication and deletion of 13q: study of a family presenting with bilateral retinoblastomas. Clin Genet 15:332–345

Rivera H, Turleau C, de Grouchy J, Junien C, Despoisses S, Zücker JM (1981) Retinoblastoma-del (13q14): report of two patients, one with a trisomic sib due to maternal insertion. Gene Dosage effect for esterase D. Hum Genet 59:211–214

Schappert-Kimmijser J, Hemmes GD, Nijland R (1966) The heredity of retinoblastoma. Ophthalmologica 151:197–213

Scheffer H, te Meerman GJ, Kruize YCM, van den Berg AHM, Penninga DP, Tan KEWP, der Kinderen DJ, Buys CHCM (1989) Linkage analysis of families with hereditary retinoblastoma: non-penetrance of mutation, revealed by combined use of markers within and flanking the Rb1 gene. Am J Hum Genet 45:252–260

Sorsby A (1972) Bilateral retinoblastoma: a dominantly inherited affection. Br Med J 2:580–583

Sparkes RS, Murphree AL, Lingua RW, Sparkes MC, Field LL, Funderburk SJ, Benedict WF (1983) Gene for hereditary retinoblastoma assigned to human chromosome 13 by linkage analysis of esterase D. Science 219:971–973

Strong LC, Riccardi VM, Ferrell RE, Sparkes RS (1981) Familial retinoblastoma and chromosome 13 deletion transmitted via an insertional translocation. Science 213:1501–1503

Tucker DP, Streinberg AG, Cogan DG (1957) Frequency of genetic transmission of sporadic retinoblastoma. Arch Ophthalmol 57:532–535

Turleau C, de Grouchy J, Chavin-Colin F, Despoisses S, Leblanc A (1983) Two cases of del(13q)-
    retinoblastoma and two cases of partial trisomy due to familial insertion. Ann Genet 26:158–160
Vogel F (1957) Neue Untersuchungen zur Genetik des Retinoblastoms. Z mensch Vererb u Konstit
    Lehre 34:205–236
Vogel F (1979) Genetics of retinoblastoma. Hum Genet 52:1–54
Vogel F, Rathenberg R (1975) Spontaneous mutation in man. Adv Hum Genet 5:223–318
Zhu X, Dunn JM, Phillips RA, Goddard AD, Paton KE, Becker A, Gallie BL (1989) Preferential
    germline mutation of the paternal allele in retinoblastoma. Nature 340:312–313

Genetic Epidemiology of Cancer and Predisposing Lesions*

L.A. CANNON-ALBRIGHT[1], D.T. BISHOP[2], D.E. GOLDGAR[3], and M.H. SKOLNICK[3]

Introduction

The common contribution of genetic factors to the susceptibility to common cancer is not well understood and not generally accepted. Although familial clustering of common cancers has been observed, only a minority of cases provide obvious support for an inherited component, and few family studies of random common cancers have been implemented. Only in rare syndromes such as Gardner's syndrome, familial adenomatous polyposis, Wilm's tumor, and retinoblastoma has the contribution of an inherited susceptibility to the etiology of cancer been confirmed.

One of the most promising approaches for understanding cancer etiology and for creating an effective cancer control program is through identification of individuals who are genetically predisposed to cancer. The genetic study of common cancers has often focused on unusual families with high penetrance. However, most individuals with cancer at common sites do not belong to such families; they either occur in smaller clusters of "familial cancer" or are solitary. A susceptibility to a premalignant lesion, which itself carried only an increased probability of conversion to malignancy, might explain why some cancers appear to cluster only rarely in families and are most often solitary. The study of the inheritance of these premalignant lesions and their associated cancers may clarify the role of inherited factors in at least a portion of cancers previously thought to be non-genetic. This may also provide an explanation for the observed familiality of some cancers in the absence of clear segregation. We hypothesize that a subset of the population carry precursor lesions, which reflect a predisposition to initiation events which lead to malignancy. These predispositions tend to be site-specific and the precursor lesions appear to be related to growth abnormalities of a particular cell type. We have studied three cancer sites which have shown strong familiality and have recognizable and identifiable precursor lesions which are apparently present for many years before overt cancer develops. We

* This research was supported by NIH grants CA-28854, CA-48711, CA-42014, CN-55428, RR-64, CA-41591, AM-35378, CA40641, and CA-36362
[1] Division of Hematology/Oncology, Department of Internal Medicine, University of Utah School of Medicine, Salt Lake City, UT, USA
[2] Genetic Epidemiology Laboratory, Imperial Cancer Research Fund, Leeds, United Kingdom
[3] Department of Medical Informatics, University of Utah School of Medicine, Salt Lake City, UT, USA

H.T. Lynch and P. Tautu (Eds.)
Recent Progress
in the Genetic Epidemiology of Cancer
© Springer-Verlag Berlin Heidelberg 1991

describe here our general approach to the genetic epidemiology of cancer and cancer precursors through a discussion of our studies of colon cancer, melanoma, and breast cancer.

Starting with genealogical records kept by the Utah Genealogical Society, we have constructed a genealogy of 1.5 million Utah descendants of pioneers (Skolnick 1980). These genealogy records have been linked to the Utah State Cancer Registry records kept in Utah since 1962 and the combined records make up the Utah Population Database.

A study of cancer in this population is advantageous because of its large, stable Mormon population and the availability of the statewide cancer records. Several unique aspects of this population are especially important in genetic studies: early polygamy, high fertility, and computerized genealogy. Utah Mormons have more than twice as many children as the US average (Skolnick et al. 1978). We have demonstrated that this population has typical Northern European gene frequencies (McLellan et al. 1984) and normal levels of inbreeding (Jorde and Skolnick 1981). Both of these characteristics are due to the British, Scandinavian, and German origin of the approximately 10 000 founders (Skolnick 1980). For most cancer sites the age-adjusted incidence rates are lower in Utah than the rates observed in the USA (Cancer in Utah 1988).

Together, these characteristics make this population appropriate for inferences about cancer etiology in populations of Northern European descent. This population has been highly cooperative with our medical studies, giving us high compliance rates. We have over 85% compliance for flexible sigmoidoscopy in our colon cancer studies, 98% compliance for nevus biopsy in our melanoma studies, and 90% compliance for four quadrant fine needle aspiration in our breast cancer studies. These compliance figures include relatives as well as spouse controls who are not at increased risk for the cancer being studied.

This unique database in Utah has allowed an analysis of the kinship of cancer cases in this well-defined population. Analysis of kinship by site showed that there is increased familiality observed for almost all cancer sites, at both close and very distant degrees of relationship (Cannon et al. 1982; Hill 1980; Skolnick et al. 1981; Bishop and Skolnick 1984). These results in combination with the long recognized increased risk of cancer in first degree relatives of cases (Skolnick et al. 1981; Woolf 1958; Macklin 1960; Lovett 1976; Anderson 1980) suggest an underlying genetic susceptibility to most cancer sites, and that there are many distantly related cases of cancer for which a commonly inherited component may be responsible.

However, even with this evidence for underlying genetic susceptibility, any attempt to study the genetic epidemiology of cancer is made difficult by late age onset, sex specificity of some cancers, and competing causes of death, all of which may censor information. Our model of cancer etiology hypothesizes a predisposing gene for precursor lesions which themselves have a relatively low probability of conversion to malignancy. The cancers themselves therefore do not demonstrate a clear mendelian pattern, but the cancer susceptibility (exhibited by the lesions) does have an inherited basis. We hypothesize precursor lesions for many cancer sites and recognize the value such markers of cancer risk hold for clarifying the genetic etiology of cancer.

An increased incidence of both the cancer and the associated lesions in certain families (higher than population rates), in combination with an observed segregation pattern, suggests a model in which some or all of the steps are genetic of familial. Current models of carcinogenesis proposed by Knudson (Knudson 1971; Knudson and Strong 1972) and extended by Moolgavkar (1978) allow for at least two rare events leading to the transformation of normal cells to malignant cells. In experimental carcinogenesis, at least three stages can be identified for transformation of a normal into a malignant cell: (i) initiation, (ii) promotion, and (iii) progression (to malignancy). The transition between these stages can be enhanced or inhibited by different agents. Weinstein et al. (1983) suggest multiple transforming genes may be necessary in the conversion of normal cells to tumor cells; these include genes related to immortalization, morphologic and growth properties, invasion, metastasis, and drug resistance. In these models the development of cancer appears to be a late or even final step in a sequence of events including biochemical, genetic, and biological changes. They postulate that origination and maintenance of a malignancy requires multiple cellular genes and changes in genomic structure and function. The steps may include the appearance of new cells with altered phenotypes, and the expansion of some altered cells to a collection, such as a polyp or a nevus. These collections of altered cells may disappear or they may persist and become sites for further cellular changes resulting in malignancy.

It is hypothesized that in hereditary cancer the initial alteration, or a susceptibility to it, is inherited, and only promotion and progression are required for lesion appearance and malignancy. The model for hereditary cases suggests that the primary event is a mutation in a gene occurring in an ancestral germ cell and inherited by the gene carriers. Mutation of the same gene on the homologous chromosome in a somatic cell would then lead to malignancy. Not all cells transform into a lesion, which suggests that in genetically predisposed individuals, although all cells may have an increased susceptibility to initiation, only some cells experience the necessary change(s) resulting in lesions. Genetic predisposition to the formation of precursor lesions could determine which cells become initiated and how many cells are initiated.

Results

Colon Cancer and Adenomatous Polyps

The adenoma/colorectal cancer association is well supported both by the evidence of the appearance of adenomatous polyps adjacent to or as part of colorectal tumors, as well as the virtually 100% risk of colorectal cancer among individuals with inherited polyp syndromes such as Gardner's syndrome or familial adenomatous polyposis (FAP). In our study (Burt et al. 1985; Cannon-Albright et al. 1988), we hypothesized that susceptibility to adenomatous polyps was inherited and that this inherited susceptibility could account for the familial clustering frequently observed among cases of colorectal cancer. Over 300 asymptomatic members of a large pedigree were studied. This pedigree was ascertained for three close relatives with colorectal cancer. The analysis demonstrated an inherited susceptibility to adenomatous polyps and colorectal cancers in this large kindred (Burt et al. 1985), and the initial observation of inherited susceptibility in this single pedigree was subsequently confirmed by studying 33 additional pedigrees (Cannon-Albright et al. 1988). These analyses suggest that an inherited susceptibility to adenomas is common, is 60% penetrant by age 80, and is responsible for the majority of colorectal cancers and adenomas observed.

The majority of colon polyps and cancers are thought to arise from environmental factors, probably dietary. Because adenomas are the precursors of colorectal cancer, a common inherited susceptibility for polyps suggests a model in which colon cancers arise from environmental (or other genetic) factors acting on polyps in individuals with an inherited predisposition. This model is graphically depicted in Fig. 1 which demonstrates how genetic or environmental factors may interact with an inherited predisposition at one of many stages on the progression to malignancy.

Melanoma

Cutaneous melanoma (CM) has been associated with an inherited cutaneous phenotype, the dysplastic nevus syndrome (DNS). This condition is characterized

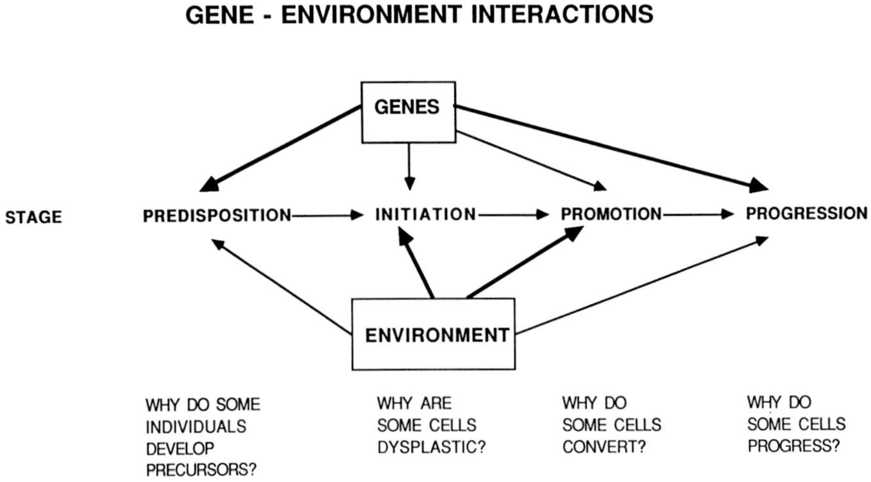

Fig. 1. Hypothesized model of the role of inherited predispositions in cancer etiology

by an increased number of nevi which are often large, and clinically and pathologically abnormal. However, there is considerable variation of phenotype within families, making diagnosis difficult. Studies of high-risk melanoma kindreds have suggested that dysplastic nevi are the precursors for melanoma in these kindreds and that such nevi can occur in high or low frequency in at-risk individuals. Studies of high-risk melanoma families suggest that dysplastic nevi are in fact very common and that the degree of dysplasia of a nevus is not related to its size or its degree of clinical atypia (Piepkorn et al. 1989); this view has been further supported by Black and Hunt (1990). These studies indicate that the melanoma precursor trait may be related to high total area of nevi and may be exhibited in at-risk individuals either as a high number of nevi or in a lower number of large nevi. An increased number of nevi has been recognized as being associated with increased risk of melanoma (Holly et al. 1987; Swerdlow et al. 1986). Clinical and histopathological dysplasia are important in that they may be representative of those particular nevi more likely to be promoted to malignancy.

We have studied high-risk melanoma families and have measured total nevus area by body location for relatives and spouses. Probands and their blood relatives had significantly more total nevi than spouses. Preliminary pedigree analysis of total nevus area suggests autosomal co-dominant inheritance of a single locus allele in high-risk melanoma pedigrees. Our further analysis of total nevus area adjusted for body surface area suggests that the most parsimonious two-locus model is a common recessive locus for high nevus count and a co-dominant locus for nevus growth which acts as a growth suppressor in one homozygote, a growth activator of equal effect in the other, and neutral in the heterozygote (unpublished data). It is not yet clear whether this two-locus model is appropriate or, for example, whether a one-locus model with interacting environmental factors underlies the observations.

Breast Cancer and Proliferative Breast Disease

Several cohort studies have demonstrated that women with proliferative breast disease (PBD) have an increased risk of developing breast cancer when compared to women with non-proliferative breast lesions and other benign breast disorders (Dupont and Page 1985; Carter et al. 1988). In these studies proliferative breast disease was diagnosed in cytological material from suspicious breast masses provided through fine-needle aspiration (FNA). We have recently extended this technique, using multiple FNAs of all four breast quadrants, in an attempt to detect the precancerous lesions of PBD (ductal hyperplasia and atypical ductal hyperplasia) in breasts without masses.

In the FNA procedure a 22-gauge needle is inserted into each quadrant of the breast and the needle is repeatedly directed for approximately eight passes to broadly sample a given quadrant. All biopsies are reviewed and histologically segregated into proliferative and non-proliferative lesions utilizing the classification scheme and criteria proposed by Dupont and Page (1985) and Page et al. (1985). We have performed random FNA of the breast in relatives of breast cancer cases and in controls. We have evaluated 68 first degree relatives of sister-sister probands and 28 controls (women marrying into these families, but not genetically related). Dupont and Page (1985) originally defined PBD diagnosed from breast mass lesions as the presence of one or more benign or atypical hyperplastic epithelial fragments. Using this definition we found six of 28 controls had PBD. This high frequency in controls suggests that the definition of the precursor needs refinement: perhaps to the presence of several hyperplastic epithelial fragments, or to the presence of multiple epithelial fragments of any type. When three or more atypical fragments are required, the frequency in controls is three out of 28 and a significant difference is noted between controls and relatives (unpublished data).

Preliminary pedigree analysis utilizing the classic definition of PBD in 17 pedigrees of sister-sister or mother-daughter pairs with breast cancer provides evidence for a dominant major gene for the combined PBD/breast cancer trait. We have refined the trait as suggested above, requiring a minimum of three such atypical fragments, and similar, stronger evidence for the dominant model is found. Figure 2 shows a breast cancer pedigree selected for two sisters with breast cancer in which proliferative breast disease was found to be present in first degree relatives using four-quadrant FNA.

Methodology

An important aspect of the study of common cancers is the ascertainment of families for study. In our studies a variety of families are chosen with different selection schemes. A careful record is kept of the reason each family was selected for study. We select "cluster" families with a specified number of relatives of a

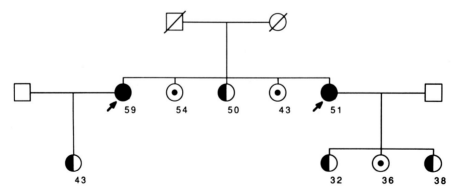

Fig. 2. Breast cancer family 1904. *Full shading* indicates breast cancer cases, original breast cancer probands are indicated with *arrows*. *Half shading* indicates presence of proliferative breast disease (PBD). *Dot* indicates screened individuals with PBD absent. Age at breast cancer or screening is indicated for all females

certain type from clinical files or the computerized genealogy, such as sister-sister pairs of breast cancer. These are chosen from the set of all possible breast cancer cases. In addition we study a set of families of "unselected" probands with the cancer of interest. These probands are selected at random from the Utah Cancer Registry with no knowledge of family history. Finally, as spouses marrying into the above families are seen, we select spouses "affected" with the "at-risk" phenotype and study their relatives. Each type of family seen provides an important piece of data. The cluster families increase the chance that, in the presence of heterogeneity, we will find families exhibiting the inherited precursor; in addition they are useful for linkage studies. By observing the frequency of the inherited precursor in the relatives of the unselected cancer probands we obtain an estimate of the percent of all individuals with the cancer of interest which are due to the inherited susceptibility. Finally, studying the families of affected spouses helps to estimate the population gene frequency as well as the percent of individuals with the at-risk phenotype who also have inherited the gene (sporadic rate). Sampling of relatives includes all first degree relatives of probands and extends to all first degree relatives of any individuals found to have the at-risk phenotype. This sampling strategy is followed to avoid bias introduced by directed sampling (Cannings and Thompson 1977).

Pedigree analysis is the primary tool used to test the hypotheses of an inherited susceptibility, as well as to estimate the associated parameters of the model and to estimate an individual's probability of carrying the hypothesized susceptibility allele. Through genetic modeling of the trait we estimate gene frequency, penetrance, and variable expression of the phenotypes within families. Since there will always be limitations on the inferences possible from observed pedigree data, all segregation analyses should always be considered a first step, to be followed by more detailed genetic analysis, such as linkage analysis, which can confirm the inferences made.

The overall aim of family studies of cancer is to localize the precursor loci associated with common cancers to specific chromosomes. Analysis of the precursor lesion provides us with a linkage hypothesis to test and a genetic locus to map. Candidate loci are of primary interest, general linkage searches follow these. Once a locus has been localized, a fine structure map can be developed around it. The markers which map the locus can then be used to (1) clarify the genetic model for the precursor, (2) clarify the analyses of factors which affect the expression of the precursors, and (3) lead to the isolation of abnormal DNA sequences. The genotype of individuals studied can then be used to better define the precursor phenotype, as well as to help evaluate environmental effects on both gene and non-gene carriers.

Conclusion

There probably exist premalignant lesions for a variety of other cancers. These lesions may not be so easily observed as those already recognized. In addition, other cancer sites may exhibit far fewer lesions and exhibit them far less frequently. For example, cells from organs that have less exposure to factors or agents inside or outside the body (such as to food, sunlight or hormones), those that have a lower growth rate, or those in which differentiation is complete early in life, may have less opportunity to express dysplasia. It may be that most cancers result from an inherited susceptibility for lesion precursors. However, for some a lesion stage may not be necessary, since the cell may already have some of the necessary characteristics of tumor cells and may require fewer stages for conversion to malignancy.

If the genes that are hypothesized as being responsible for melanoma, colon cancer, and breast cancer are oncogenes, they may be a new class of oncogenes. The currently known set of oncogenes appear to be transforming genes, while these appear to be predisposing genes; attempts to relate the original set of known oncogenes to these predispositions have not yet been successful.

References

Anderson DE (1980) Risk in families of patients with colon cancer. In: Winawer S, Schottenfeld D, Sherlock P (eds) Colorectal cancer: prevention, epidemiology, and screening. Raven, New York, pp 109–115

Bishop DT, Skolnick MH (1984) Genetic epidemiology of cancer in Utah genealogies: a prelude to the molecular genetics of common cancers. J Cell Physiol [Suppl] 3:63–77

Black WC, Hunt WC (1990) Histologic correlation with the clinical diagnosis of dysplastic nevus. Am J Surg Path 14:44–52

Burt RW, Bishop DT, Cannon LA, Dowdle MA, Lee RG, Skolnick MH (1985) Dominant inheritance of adenomatous colonic polyps and colorectal cancer. N Engl J Med 312:1540–1544

Cancer in Utah (1988) Statistical and epidemiological report 1973–1985. Utah Cancer Registry, Salt Lake City, Utah

Cannings C, Thompson EA (1977) Ascertainment in the sequential sampling of pedigrees. Clin Genet 12:208–212

Cannon L, Bishop DT, Skolnick M, Hunt S, Lyon JL, Smart CR (1982) Genetic epidemiology of prostate cancer in the Utah Mormon genealogy. Cancer Surv 1:47–69

Cannon-Albright LA, Skolnick MH, Bishop DT, Lee RG, Burt RW (1988) Common inheritance of susceptibility to colonic adenomatous polyps and associated colorectal cancers. N Engl J Med 319:533–537

Carter CL, Corle DK, Micozzi MS, Schatzkin A, Taylor P (1988) A prospective study of breast cancer in 16 692 women with benign breast disease. Am J Epidemiol 128:467–477

Dupont WD, Page DL (1985) Risk factors for breast cancer in women with proliferative breast disease. New Engl J Med 312:146–151

Hill J (1980) A kinship survey of cancer in the Utah Mormon population. PhD thesis, University of Utah

Holly EA, Kelly JW, Shpall SN, Chiu SH (1987) Number of melanocytic nevi as a major risk factor for malignant melanoma. J Am Acad Dermatol 17:459–468

Jorde LB, Skolnick MH (1981) Demographic and genetic application of computerized record linking: the Utah Mormon genealogy. Information et Sciences Humaines 56–57:105–117

Knudson AG (1971) Mutation and cancer: a statistical study of retinoblastoma. Proc Natl Acad Sci USA 68:820–823

Knudson AG, Strong LC (1972) Mutation and cancer: a model for Wilm's tumor of the kidney. J Natl Cancer Inst 48:313

Lovett E (1976) Family studies in cancer of the colon and rectum. Br J Surg 63:13–28

Macklin MT (1960) Inheritance of cancer of the stomach and large intestine in man. JNCI 24:551–571

McLellan T, Jorde LB, Skolnick MH (1984) Genetic distances between the Utah Mormons and related populations. Am J Hum Genet 36:836–857

Moolgavkar SH (1978) The multistage theory of carcinogenesis and the age distribution of cancer in man. JNCI 61:49–52

Page DL, Dupont WD, Rogers LW, Rados MS (1985) Atypical hyperplastic lesions of the female breast. Cancer 55:2698–2708

Piepkorn M, Meyer LJ, Goldgar D, Seuchter SA, Cannon-Albright LA, Skolnick MH, Zone JJ (1989) The dysplastic melanocytic nevus: a prevalent lesion that correlates poorly with clinical phenotype. J Am Acad Dermatol 20:407–415

Skolnick M (1980) The Utah genealogical data base: a resource for genetic epidemiology. In: Cairns J, Lyon JL, Skolnick M (eds) Banbury Report No. 4: cancer incidence in defined populations. Cold Spring Harbor Laboratory, New York, pp 285–297

Skolnick M, Bean L, May D, Arbon V, de Nevers K, Cartwright P (1978) Mormon demographic history. I. Nuptiality and fertility of once-married couples. Popul Stud 32:5–19

Skolnick M, Bishop DT, Carmelli D, Gardner E, Hadley R, Hasstedt, Hill JR, Hunt S, Lyon JL, Smart CR, Williams RR (1981) A population based assessment of familial cancer risk in Utah Mormon genealogies. In: Arrighi F, Rao PN, Stubblefield E (eds) Genes, Chromosomes and Neoplasia. Raven, New York, pp 477–500

Swerdlow AJ, English J, MacKie RM, O'Doherty CJ, Hunter JAA, Clark J, Hole DJ (1986) Benign melanocytic naevi as a risk factor for malignant melanoma. Br Med J 292:1555–1559

Weinstein B, Gattoni-Celli S, Kirschmeier P, Lambert M, Hsiao W, Backer J, Jeffrey A (1983) Multistage carcinogenesis involves multiple genes and multiple mechanisms. In: Mak TW, Tannock I (eds) Cellular and Molecular Biology of Neoplasia. Liss, New York, pp 127–138

Woolf CM (1958) A genetic study of carcinoma of the large intestine in man. Am J Hum Genet 10:42–47

Search for Genetic Factors in the Etiology of Breast Cancer*

P. Devilee

Introduction

The genetic basis of cancer has in recent years evolved into a virtually undisputed concept (Weinberg 1989). The idea that cancer is engendered by changes in the genetic make-up of a somatic cell still forms the premises of numerous — if not all — molecular-genetic cancer research projects. Many of these have been aimed at identifying the targets of the changes, i.e., which are the genes that upon their structural alteration become intimately involved in the tumorigenic process? This has led to the discovery of a large group of genes, collectively addressed as oncogenes. More recently, mainly through cell fusion studies (Harris 1988) and work on hereditary retinoblastoma (Knudson 1989), another class of genes has been identified, termed antioncogenes or, more appropriately, tumor suppressor genes. The finding that a genetic change as little as a single point-mutation can distinguish the normal constitutional homologue of c-Ha-*ras* from its tumorigenic counterpart (Bos 1989) still stands as a paradigm for the role of gene mutation in tumorigenesis.

Breast Cancer

Progress in characterizing breast cancer in genetic terms has been relatively slow, especially when compared with hematopoietic malignancies. This may be due to the complex biology and growth characteristics of the tumor on the one hand, and to the long lack of appropriate technology on the other. Along with the advent of better cytogenetic and molecular tools for genetic analysis, some major contributions in this field are emerging and others may be expected in the near future. I will briefly review here two strategies followed in our own laboratory. These are: (i) interphase cytogenetics, and (ii) the screening for chromosome regions undergoing loss of heterozygosity in the tumor. It is apparent that DNA flow

* The author is supported by the Royal Dutch Cancer Society (Koningin Wilhelmina Fonds, Grant No. 1KW 87-15

Department of Human Genetics, University of Leiden, Wassenaarseweg 72, 2333 AL Leiden, The Netherlands

H.T. Lynch and P. Tautu (Eds.)
Recent Progress
in the Genetic Epidemiology of Cancer
© Springer-Verlag Berlin Heidelberg 1991

cytometry as well as karyotyping will not be able to identify genetic entities involved in breast cancer. The former because it has too limited a genetic resolution, the latter because the abundant presence of undefined marker chromosomes greatly obscures the detection of any specific genetic aberration, if at all visible at the cytogenetic level. It would at least require large series of tumors to be investigated, a requirement which is notoriously difficult to meet in the case of breast cancer.

In Situ Hybridization: Interphase Cytogenetics

Interphase cytogenetics by non-radioactive in situ hybridization (ISH) methods may be able to render virtually all cells isolated from a breast tumor amenable for cytogenetic analysis, regardless of which phase of the cell cycle they are in. The development of this technique was boosted a few years ago by the development of a number of repetitive DNA probes, which were able to specifically detect the centromeric or heterochromatic regions of particular chromosomes. Single-copy DNA probes in the order of 1-3 kb are generally unproductive when applied in a non-radioactive ISH on metaphase spreads as well as on interphase nuclei. By contrast, chromosome-specific repetitive DNA sequences generate bright fluorescence signals on cognate chromosomes, and the target sequences can also be easily visualized in the interphase nucleus. The resulting number of spots revealed per nucleus was shown to reflect the number of chromosomes present therein (Fig. 1; Cremer et al. 1986). A cloned representative of the alpha-satellite DNA family on chromosome 18, designated L1.84 (Devilee et al. 1986), successfully led to detection of a trisomy 18 in cells obtained from an amniotic-fluid cell culture after amniocentesis at the 17th week of pregnancy (Cremer et al. 1986). The majority of nuclei ($> 90\%$) contained three spots/nucleus (S/N) after ISH with L1.84, whereas preparations of normal diploid nuclei obtained from fibroblasts or peripheral white blood cells of healthy donors typically revealed two S/N in $> 85\%$ of the nuclei examined. This approach can be applied to any chromosome for which a suitable repetitive DNA sequence is available. At present, this implies that approximately two-thirds of the total human chromosome complement (Table 1) is amenable for analysis of numerical abnormalities in interphase cells.

Detection of Chromosome Abnormalities in Tumors

The correlation between the presence of chromosome abnormalities, as evidence by cytogenetic analysis, and a deviant number of S/N after ISH, has been demonstrated on several tumor cell lines (Cremer et al. 1988; Devilee et al. 1988; Hopman et al. 1988). In the majority of nuclei prepared from MCF7, a cell line established from a pleural effusion from a breast cancer patient, three S/N were noted after ISH with probe PUC1.77 (Devilee et al. 1988), which specifically

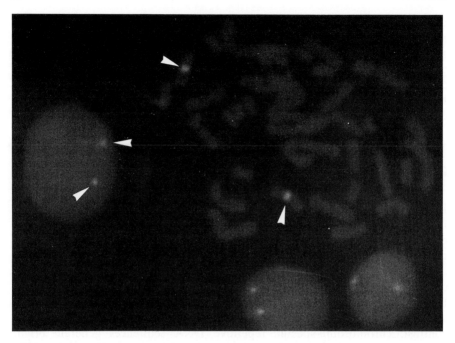

Fig. 1. In situ hybridization of probe pHUR98 (Table 1), which detects the heterochromatic region of chromosome 9 (Moyzis et al. 1987), to a lymphocyte metaphase spread obtained from a healthy donor. Following avidin-FITC treatment, heterochromatic regions of both chromosome 9 homologs stain brightly (*arrow heads*), while interphase nuclei each contain two distinct spots (exemplified by *arrow heads* in one nucleus). Propidium-iodine counterstaining. (Our unpublished results)

detects the heterochromatic region of chromosome 1 (Cremer et al. 1988). In metaphase spreads of MCF-7, the probe identified three chromosomes, one of which, however, was clearly a derivative chromosome 1 showing a large deletion that involved most of the long arm (Devilee et al. 1988). More recently, a close comparison of GTG-banding and ISH methods with eight different repetitive sequences applied to metaphases isolated from two different ovarian carcinoma cell lines indicated that the target sequences of some probes can be visualized on cytogenetically undefineable marker chromosomes (Smit et al. in press). This illustrates one of the shortcomings of the use of centromeric repetitive DNA: a deviant number of S/N does not per se indicate a numerical change of the complete chromosome which is detected by the probe.

The target sites of repetitive probes specific for the centromeric regions of chromosomes 1 and 18 have been detected in freshly isolated interphase nuclei of carcinomas of the breast (Devilee et al. 1988) and bladder (Hopman et al. 1988). We are currently also applying probes detecting the centromeric regions of chromosomes 7, 11, and 17. Together, these studies provide an indication of the potentialities and drawbacks of the approach. The most important impact of interphase cytogenetics of solid tumors will be the increasing knowledge of

Table 1. Chromosome-specific repetitive DNA probes and their use in interphase cytogenetics

Chrom.	Name	Rep. fam.	Copy no.	Specificity[a]	Utility[b]
1	PUC1.77	Sat. III	?	Very Good	Good
1p36	D1Z2	Unknown	?	Good	Good
3	D3Z1	Alphoid	~ 500	Good	Not tested
4	pGXba11	Alphoid	~ 3000	Medium	Not tested
6	D6Z1	Alphoid	?	Good	Good
7	D7Z1	Alphoid	?	Good	Good
8	D8Z2	Alphoid	?	Not tested	Not tested
9	pHUR98	Sat. III	?	Good	Good
10	D10Z1	Alphoid	~ 250	Good	Good
11	D11Z1	Alphoid	~ 500	Medium	Medium
12	pα12H8	Alphoid	~ 5000	Good	Good
15	D15Z1	Sat. III	~ 3000	Good	Good
16	pHUR195	Sat. II	?	Good	Good
16	pSE16	Alphoid	?	Medium	Medium
17	D17Z1	Alphoid	~ 500	Very good	Good
18	D18Z1	Alphoid	~ 2000	Good	Good
20	D20Z1	Alphoid	~ 100	Good	Not tested
22	D22Z3	Unknown	~ 5000	Good	Medium
X	DXZ1	Alphoid	~ 5000	Good	Not tested
Y	DYZ1	Sat. III	?	Good	Good

[a] Under high-stringency hybridization conditions: "very good" when no hybridization to other chromosomes can be seen; "good" when there is a weak inconsistent cross-hybridization with other chromosomes; "medium" when the probe is persistently showing minor cross-hybridizing signals on other chromosomes

[b] Generally dependent on the specificity of hybridization. "Good" when spots/nucleus can be easily visualized and counted. "Medium" when cross-hybridizing minor binding-sites interfere with the proper evaluation of spots

cytogenetic intratumor heterogeneity. This heterogeneity has been observed in both solid tumors and tumor cell lines and is indicated by the presence of significant populations of nuclei carrying a distinct number of S/N (Fig. 2). Notably, in many cases the heterogeneity with respect to S/N content of the nuclei is not seen in DNA flow cytometry, in which a single peak is formed. The fact that a 25% admixture of cells with a trisomy 18 to normal diploid cells could be reliably detected after ISH with probe L1.84 (Devilee et al. 1988) is of direct relevance for the significance of the observed heterogeneity in tumors. Characterization of a solid tumor with a broad set of DNA probes to generate a chromosome profile will provide more detailed insight into its cytogenetic complexity. This may be particularly worthwhile for those cases in which lymph-node metastases can be compared with the primary tumor.

Interphase Cytogenetics: Future Applications

Interphase cytogenetics in its present state allows only the identification of numerical changes in the centromeric regions of particular chromosomes in the

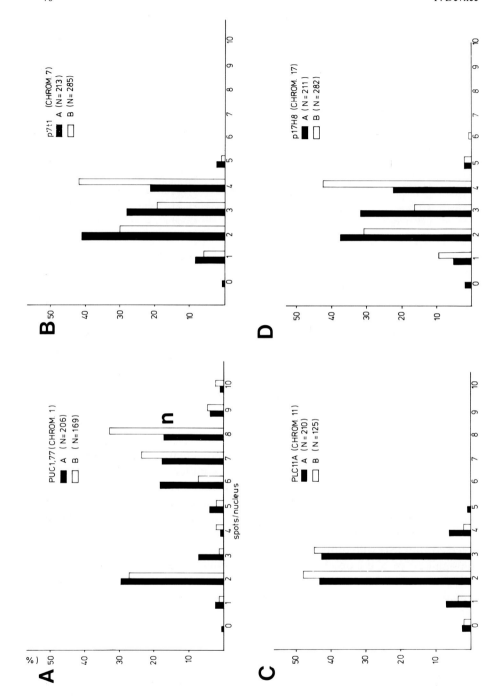

interphase nucleus. It is not yet able to reveal structural abnormalities of the chromosomes that are detected. However, several developments may ultimately create favorable conditions to meet this requirement. One of these is based on the introduction of a number of different chemical modifications for probe sequences in conjunction with three different fluorochromes. This allows the hybridization of two, three, or even more probes simultaneously and their detection as distinctly colored signals in fluorescence microscopy (Nederlof et al. 1989). This will substantially speed up the characterization of nuclei isolated from tumors by a large set of probes, and also give further insight into the cytogenetic heterogeneity of that tumor. More important, however, is that bi-color ISH performed with selected pools of cloned single-copy sequences potentially allows the identification of specific translocation events in the interphase nucleus, provided that the two pools flank the translocation break point (Cremer et al. 1986). Recently, a pool of 32 single-copy inserts, comprising 94 kb from human chromosome region 21q22.3, was demonstrated to be capable of detecting by non-radioactive ISH a trisomy chromosome 21 in interphase nuclei obtained from Down syndrome (47, + 21) individuals (Lichter et al. 1988). Thus, particular chromosomal bands can be visualized in the interphase nucleus. No combination of two appropriate plasmid pools is as yet available for the detection of any of the important translocations occurring in human tumors. However, the combined use of two repetitive DNA probes, one detecting the heterochromatic region of chromosome 1 and the other detecting band 1p36, has been able to identify breakage events on the short arm of chromosome 1 (Van Dekken and Bauman 1988). A modified procedure exploits a complete genomic DNA library cloned from a flow-cytometry-sorted human chromosome. Ubiquitous repetitive sequences present in the library are reannealed with an excess of unlabeled total human DNA prior to applying the probe to metaphase spreads or interphase nuclei for ISH. This procedure has been termed suppression or competition hybridization and results in a specific fluorescent staining of the chromosome from pter to qter (Pinkel et al. 1988). "Chromosome painting" has general applications for the delineation of complex chromosome translocations in metaphase spreads (Pinkel et al. 1988). For interphase cytogenetics of nuclei derived from solid tumors, the use of defined plasmid pools is preferable, since the detected chromosome region will then be revealed as a distinct spot, as opposed to the blurred pattern of staining of a chromosome domain that is achieved when a complete library is used. Alternatively, large human DNA fragments of up to 800 kb contained in yeast artificial chromosomes or a small set of overlapping cosmid clones may prove to be valuable substitutes for plasmid pools. Principally,

Fig. 2A-D. Histograms of spots/nucleus distributions obtained independently by two observers *A* and *B*. Nuclei from the same breast tumor were hybridized in situ with each of four different repetitive DNA probes specific for the centromeric regions of chromosomes 1 (**A**), 7 (**B**), 11 (**C**), and 17 (**D**). The tumor was multiploid in DNA flow cytometry (DNA indices of 1.67 and 1.83) and contained approximately 60% tumor cells. (Our unpublished results)

this would allow the detection of deletions in interphase nuclei, with the advantage of obtaining important information on the intratumor heterogeneity of this genetic defect. By selecting cosmid clones that favorably cover the region of interest it should be feasible to detect interstitial microdeletions (Trask et al. 1989).

Finally, non-radioactive ISH protocols utilizing peroxidase for hybrid detection have enabled the detection of chromosome target sites in tissue sections (Emmerich et al. 1989) which may be prepared either from frozen or paraffin-embedded tissue. Thus, chromosome aneuploidy can be studied within the context of a variety of histological and morphological parameters, and the question whether the progression of the tumor has given rise to cytogenetically distinct foci of cells becomes amenable for analysis.

Loss of Heterozygosity in Breast Cancer

A general characteristic of tumor cells is the loss of the accuracy of chromosome disjunction, which usually leads to under- or overrepresentation of particular chromosomes or parts thereof, relative to the normal diploid genome. It has been hypothesized that chromosome aneuploidy may allow malignant cells to express particular recessive phenotypes (Ohno 1974; Klein 1981) while the role of gene dosage in the initiation and propagation of genetic instability has recently also been emphasized (Holliday 1989). In cancer studies it is therefore important to be able to distinctly mark each homologue of a chromosome pair so as to investigate their involvement in nondisjunctional or deletion events. The impact of restriction fragment length polymorphisms (RFLPs) to cancer research has been demonstrated by work on retinoblastoma (Cavenee et al. 1983). Here the first tumor in which the phenomenon of loss of constitutional heterozygosity was observed on the long arm of chromosome 13. Eventually this led to the identification of a predisposing tumor suppressor gene (Knudson 1989). In families with hereditary retinoblastoma, DNA polymorphisms within the gene were shown to be linked with the disease and to represent valuable markers for risk estimations (Wiggs et al. 1988).

Breast cancer may also occur in a number of different hereditary forms (Go et al. 1983; Lynch et al. 1984). Furthermore, loss of heterozygosity (LOH) has also been observed on various chromosomes in malignancies other than retinoblastoma, including some without a familial component (Green 1988). Analogous to the retinoblastoma situation, allele losses in these tumors are generally taken as hallmarks of chromosome regions harboring tumor suppressor genes (Green 1988). Therefore it seems reasonable to investigate whether LOH is involved in breast cancer development. Since it may be inferred that chromosomes undergoing frequent allele loss in the tumor may also harbor genes involved in the genetic predisposition to breast cancer, the identification of these regions may have important impact for family studies.

Concurrent LOH at Multiple Loci in Breast Cancer

Several studies have been aimed at delineating the chromosome regions involved in LOH in breast tumors (Table 2). To date, none of these has investigated tumor genotypes at all possible chromosome arms (allelotype, for terminology, see Vogelstein et al. 1989). Therefore, the matter of specificity of the reported allele losses is still largely indeterminate. This may explain why some of the earlier reports are in conflict in this regard. Ali et al. (1987) find allele losses in region 11p15 in approximately 20% of the informative cases, and virtually no LOH on five other chromosomes, including 13q. By contrast, Lundberg et al. (1987) find the highest frequency of LOH (25%) occurring on 13q, and no evidence for the involvement of 11p15. A role for the retinoblastoma gene in breast carcinoma is strongly implicated by the finding that it is rearranged in some primary tumors (T'Ang et al. 1988; Devilee et al. 1989), leading to loss of expression (Varley et al. 1989). More recent studies have hinted at more complex patterns of allele loss in breast tumors. Mackay et al. (1988a,b) have noted LOH to occur on 11p15 as well as on 17p in a consecutive series of 100 tumors. Four chromosomal regions, including 3p, 11p15, 13q, and 17p (Fig. 3), were found to be involved in LOH in a series of 64 breast tumors (Devilee et al. 1989). With a total of merely ten chromosome arms investigated in this study, about one-third of the tumors showed concurrent LOH on two to four different chromosomes. We have meanwhile extended this to 15 chromosome arms, covering approximately 50% of the total genome, and have found allelic imbalance at loci on chromosomes 1q and 6 in ~ 50%–60% of informative cases. Multiple allele loss is noted in about half the tumors (Devilee et al., unpublished data). The involvement of 1q in LOH was recently also found by Chen et al. (1989). Interestingly, all chromosomes thus far observed to undergo LOH relatively frequently in breast tumors (Table 2) have been found to be similarly involved in other tumors (Green 1988). Concurrent LOH at a number of different loci seems rather common, as it has also been noted

Table 2. Allele losses in primary breast tumors

Reference	1p	1q	3p	5q	6	11p	13q	14q	17p	17q
						Chromosome region				
Theillet et al. 1986						**				
Lundberg et al. 1987							**	*	*	
Ali et al. 1987						**				**
Mackay et al. 1988a				*		**				
Mackay et al. 1988b									***	
Genuardi et al. 1989	**									
Devilee et al. 1989			***			**	**		***	**
Devilee et al. unpubl.	*	**			***					
Chen et al. 1989		**								

* LOH in 5%–20%; ** LOH in 20%–50%; *** LOH in > 50%; observed in at least five formative cases

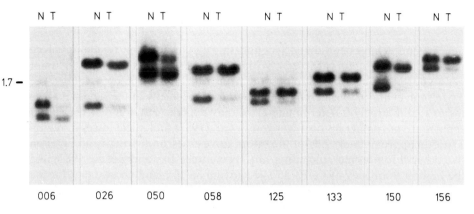

Fig. 3. Southern blot analysis of matching normal (lymphocyte) DNA (*N*) and tumor DNA (*T*) of eight breast cancer patients with probe pYNZ22.1 (D17S5), which has been assigned to the short arm of chromosome 17. Case numbers are below each pair of lanes. Number to the *left* indicates the constant band detected by D17S5 in kilobases. All patients are constitutionally heterozygous at this locus, while one allele is lost in their tumor through somatic events. In some cases, a faint residual band can be seen in the tumor, which may be ascribed either to contaminating normal DNA derived from stromal cells or infiltrating lymphocytes, or to tumor cell heterogeneity. (Reprinted from Genomics 5: pp 554–560, 1989)

in carcinoma of the colon (Vogelstein et al. 1989), lung (Yokota et al. 1987), and osteosarcoma (Toguchida et al. 1988). The question that arises is whether all these chromosome regions contain tumor suppressor genes. A candidate target gene for the deletions on chromosome 17p is the oncogene p53 (Baker et al. 1989) which was recently also ascribed tumor-suppressive functions (Finlay et al. 1989). However, the fact that in most tumors with 17p deletions the remaining p53 allele is point-mutated and actively expressed (Nigro et al. 1989) suggests a genetic mechanism distinct from that operating on the retinoblastoma gene. Indeed, no genetic linkage with 17p markers flanking p53 has been detected in families with excess breast cancer or colorectal carcinoma.

Perhaps it is not surprising to find so many chromosomes involved in LOH in view of the complex cytogenetic changes observed in most solid tumors, together with a high degree of aneuploidy as measured by DNA flow cytometry. It has been suggested that the maintenance of the genetic integrity of a normal diploid cell depends on the presence of two copies of specific genes (Holliday 1989). A change in gene dosage of one or more of these genes may trigger a general loss of accuracy in chromosome segregation at mitosis, leading to a so-called chromosome error propagation. According to this hypothesis, it seems likely that a fair number of losses are random events, as a result of this genetic instability. Each tumor may be expected to be unique in its genotypic diversification characteristics. However, if we assume that a majority of the chromosomes showing more or less frequent LOH contain genes whose product concentration in the nucleus or cytoplasm means a critical factor in determining the cell's phenotype, then the concurrent LOH at multiple loci is not without biological consequence for the progression and clinical behavior of the tumor.

Allele Loss in Breast Cancer: Biological Meaning

Will it be possible to discriminate between the genetic events that are rate-limiting for breast cancer development and those that are merely associated with progression? Whatever the biological implication of concurrent allelic losses, the phenomenon largely obscures the identification of tumor-predisposing entities such as they are defined by Knudson's theory (Knudson 1989). Nevertheless, the concept proposed by Knudson justifies attempts to connect allele loss with genetic predisposition in breast cancer families. We should be aware, however, that absence of genetic linkage to a region that is often deleted in tumors does not preclude the role of this chromosomal change in tumor development. The situation regarding colorectal cancer is instructive in this matter: a predisposing gene is located on the long arm of chromosome 5, while deletions in the tumor are often found on 17p and 18q. A first achievement in the study of breast cancer must therefore be the compilation of a complete allelotype of a fair number of tumors in order to identify the chromosomes involved in LOH. Further, the critical chromosomal regions should be delineated as accurately as possible, using mitotic deletion mapping. This may also lead to the identification of the target gene through reverse genetics procedures. It will become extremely important to do this in large series of tumor specimens, which should also contain rare subgroups of breast carcinomas such as hereditary tumors, male breast tumors, tumors from very young patients, and suspect precursor lesions such as atypical hyperplasias. Interphase cytogenetics may be helpful in addressing the matter of heterogeneity: if the deletion has occurred in all tumor cells, this might be taken as evidence that it represents an early rate-limiting event; if it has occurred in particular subsets of tumor cells, it might reflect a phenomenon associated with progression. When such characterizations are apparent in the hereditary tumors of one or two patients within a single, large, breast-cancer family, they could provide important clues with regard to the location of predisposing genes.

Breast cancer genetics is slowly coming of age. Several chromosomal regions and, in some instances, particular genes have been shown to undergo alterations in the tumor. Allelic deletions or chromosome imbalance are major events in breast carcinoma and may represent important mechanisms in tumor predisposition and progression. Not discussed here are oncogene activations, the most conspicuous of which in breast cancer is the amplification of c-erbB-2 or c-neu (Van de Vijver et al. 1989). Much remains to be done, however. Not only will it be necessary to identify all major genetic changes in extended series of breast tumors, but it will also become pivotal to study these changes in a multidisciplinary setting in order to understand their involvement in the complex biology of these tumors.

Acknowledgement. The critical reading of this manuscript by Dr. C.J. Cornelisse is kindly acknowledged.

References

Ali IU, Lidereau R, Theillet Ch, Callahan R (1987) Reduction to homozygosity of genes on chromosome 11 in human breast neoplasia. Science 238:185–188

Baker SJ, Fearon ER, Nigro JM, Hamilton SR, Preisinger AC, Jessup JM, Van Tuinen P, Ledbetter DH, Barker D, Nakamura Y, White R, Vogelstein B (1989) Chromosome 17 deletions and p53 gene mutations in colorectal carcinomas. Science 244:217–221

Bos JL (1989) Ras oncogenes in human cancer: a review. Cancer Res 49:4682–4689

Cavenee WK, Dryja TP, Philips RA, Benedict WF, Godbout R, Gallie BL, Murphree AL, Strong LC, White RL (1983) Expression of recessive alleles by chromosomal mechanisms in retinoblastoma. Nature 305:779–784

Chen L-C, Dollbaum C, Smith H (1989) Loss of heterozygosity on chromosome 1q in human breast cancer. Proc Natl Acad Sci USA 86:7204–7207

Cremer T, Landegent J, Bruckner A, Scholl H, Schardin M, Hager H, Devilee P, Pearson P, Van der Ploeg M (1986) Detection of chromosome aberrations in the human interphase nucleus by visualization of specific target DNAs with radioactive and non-radioactive in situ hybridization techniques: diagnosis of trisomy 18 with probe L184. Hum Genet 74:346–352

Cremer T, Tesin D, Hopman AHN, Manuelidis M (1988) Rapid interphase and metaphase assessment of specific chromosomal changes in neuroectodermal tumor cells by in situ hybridization with chemically modified DNA probes. Exp Cell Res 176:199–220

Devilee P, Cremer T, Slagboom P, Bakker E, Scholl H, Hager H, Stevenson A, Cornelisse C, Pearson P (1986) Two subsets of human alphoid repetitive DNA show distinct preferential localization in the pericentric regions of chromosomes 13, 18 and 21. Cytogenet Cell Genet 41:193–202

Devilee P, Thierry RF, Kolluri R, Hopman AHN, Williard HF, Pearson PL, Cornelisse CJ (1988) Detection of chromosome aneuploidy in interphase nuclei from human primary breast tumors using chromosome specific repetitive DNA-probes. Cancer Res 48:5825–5830

Devilee P, Van den Broek M, Kuipers-Dijkshoorn N, Kolluri R, Meera Khan P, Pearson PL, Cornelisse CJ (1989) At least four different chromosomal regions are involved in loss of heterozygosity in human breast carcinoma. Genomics 5:554–560

Emmerich P, Jauch A, Hofmann M-C, Cremer T, Walt H (1989) Interphase cytogenetics in paraffin embedded sections from human testicular germ cell tumor xenografts and in corresponding cultured cells. Lab Invest 61:235–242

Finlay CA, Hinds PW, Levine AJ (1989) The p53 proto-oncogene can act as a suppressor of transformation. Cell 57:1083–1093

Genuardi M, Tsihira H, Anderson DE, Saunders GF (1989) Distal deletion of chromosome 1p in ductal carcinoma of the breast. Am J Hum Genet 45:73–82

Go RCP, King M-C, Bailey-Wilson J, Elston RC, Lynch HT (1983) Genetic epidemiology of breast cancer and associated cancers in high-risk families. I. Segregation analysis. J Natl Cancer Inst 71:455–462

Green AR (1988) Recessive mechanisms of malignancy. Br J Cancer 58:115–121

Harris H (1988) The analysis of malignancy by cell fusion: the position in 1988. Cancer Res 48:3302–3306

Holliday R (1989) Chromosome error propagation and cancer. Trends Genet 5:42–45

Hopman AHN, Ramaekers FCS, Raap AK, Beck JLM, Devilee P, Van der Ploeg M, Vooijs GP (1988) In situ hybridization as a tool to study numerical chromosome aberrations in solid bladder tumors. Histochemistry 89:307–316

Klein G (1981) The role of gene dosage and genetic transposition in carcinogenesis. Nature 294:313–318

Knudson AG (1989) Hereditary cancers disclose a class of cancer genes. Cancer 63:1888–1891

Lichter P, Cremer T, Tang C-JC, Watkins PC, Manuelidis L, Ward DC (1988) Rapid detection of human chromosome 21 aberrations by in situ hybridization. Proc Natl Acad Sci USA 85:9664–9668

Lundberg C, Skoog L, Cavenee WK, Nordenskjold M (1987) Loss of heterozygosity in human ductal breast tumors indicates a recessive mutation on chromosome 13. Proc Natl Acad Sci USA 84:2372–2376

Lynch HT, Albano WA, Heieck JJ, Mulcahy GM, Lynch JF, Layton MA, Danes BS (1984) Genetics, biomarkers, and the control of breast cancer: a review. Cancer Genet Cytogen 13:43–92

Mackay J, Elder PA, Porteous DJ, Steel CM, Hawkins RA, Going JJ, Chetty U (1988a) Partial deletion of chromosome 11p in breast cancer correlates with size of primary tumour and oestrogen receptor level. Br J Cancer 58:710–714

Mackay J, Steel CM, Elder PA, Forrest APM, Evans HJ (1988b) Allele loss on the short arm of chromosome 17 in breast cancers. The Lancet II:1384–1385

Moyzis RK, Albright KL, Bartholdi MF, Cram LS, Deaven LL, Hildebrand CE, Joste NE, Longmire JL, Meyne J, Schwarzacher-Robinson T (1987) Human chromosome-specific repetitive DNA sequences: novel markers for genetic analysis. Chromosoma 95:375–386

Nederlof PM, Robinson D, Abuknesha R, Wiegant J, Hopman AHN, Tanke HJ, Raap AK (1989) Three-color fluorescence in situ hybridization for the simultaneous detection of multiple nucleic acid sequences. Cytometry 10:20–27

Nigro JM, Baker SJ, Preisinger AC, Jessup JM, Hostetter R, Cleary K, Bigner SH, Davidson N, Baylin S, Devilee P, Glover T, Collins FS, Weston A, Modali R, Harris CC, Vogelstein B (1989) Mutations in the p53 gene occur in diverse human tumor types. Nature 342:705–708

Ohno S (1974) Aneuploidy as a possible means employed by malignant cells to express recessive phenotypes. In: German J (ed) Chromosomes and cancer. Wiley, New York

Pinkel D, Landegent J, Collins C, Fuscoe J, Segraves R, Lucas J, Gray J (1988) Fluorescence in situ hybridization with human chromosome-specific libraries: detection of trisomy 21 and translocations of chromosome 4. Proc Natl Acad Sci USA 85:9138–9142

Smit VTHBM, Wessels JW, Mollevanger P, Schrier PI, Raap AK, Beverstock GC, Cornelisse CJ (1990) Combined GTG-banding and non-radioactive in situ hybridization improves characterization of complex karyotypes. Cytogenet Cell Genet (in press)

T'Ang A, Varley JM, Chakraborty S, Murphree AL, Fung Y-KT (1988) Structural rearrangement of the retinoblastoma gene in human breast carcinoma. Science 242:263–266

Theillet C, Lidereau R, Escot C, Hutzell P, Brunet M, Gest J, Schlom J, Callahan R (1986) Loss of a c-H-ras-1 allele and aggressive human primary breast carcinomas. Cancer Res 46:4776–4781

Toguchida J, Ishizaki K, Sasaki MS, Ikenaga M, Sugimoto M, Kotoura Y, Yamamuro T (1988) Chromosomal reorganization for the expression of recessive mutation of retinoblastoma susceptibility gene in the development of osteosarcoma. Cancer Res 48:3939–3943

Trask B, Pinkel D, Van den Engh G (1989) The proximity of DNA sequences in interphase cell nuclei is correlated to genomic distance and permits ordering of cosmids spanning 250 kilobase pairs. Genomics 5:710–717

Van Dekken H, Bauman JGJ (1988) A new application of in situ hybridization: detection of numerical and structural chromosome aberrations with a combination centromeric-telomeric DNA probe. Cytogenet Cell Genet 48:188–189

Van de Vijver MJ, Peterse JL, Mooi WJ, Lomans J, Verbruggen M, Van de Bersselaar R, Devilee P, Cornelisse C, Bos JL, Yarnold J, Nusse R (1989) Oncogene activations in human breast cancer. Cancer Cells 7:385–391

Varley JM, Armour J, Swallow JE, Jeffreys AJ, Ponder BAJ, T'Ang A, Fung Y-KT, Brammar WJ, Walker RA (1989) The retinoblastoma gene is frequently altered leading to loss of expression in primary breast tumors. Oncogene 4:725–729

Vogelstein B, Fearon ER, Kern SE, Hamilton SR, Preisinger AC, Nakamura Y, White R (1989) Allelotype of colorectal carcinomas. Science 244:207–211

Weinberg RA (1989) Oncogenes, antioncogenes, and the molecular bases of multistep carcinogenesis. Cancer Res 49:3713–3721

Wiggs J, Nordenskjøld M, Yandell D, Rapaport J, Grondin V, Janson M, Werelius B, Petersen R, Craft A, Riedel K, Liberfarb R, Walton D, Wilson W, Dryja TP (1988) Prediction of the risk of hereditary retinoblastoma, using DNA polymorphisms within the retinoblastoma gene. New Engl J Med 318:151–157

Yokota J, Wada M, Shimosato Y, Terada M, Sugimura T (1987) Loss of heterozygosity on chromosomes 3, 13, and 17 in small cell carcinoma and on chromosome 3 in adenocarcinoma of the lung. Proc Natl Acad Sci USA 84:9252–9256

Molecular, Cytogenetic and Linkage Analysis of Chromosome 11p Regions Involved in Wilms' Tumour and Associated Congenital Diseases*

M. Mannens[1], J. Hoovers[1], E.M. Bleeker-Wagemakers[2], J. Bliek[1], B. Redeker[1], R. John[3], P. Little[3], P.A. Voûte[4], C. Heyting[1*], R.M. Slater[1], and A. Westerveld[1]

Congenital Deletions Associated with Human Tumours

Congenital deletions associated with human tumours have been described for retinoblastoma (chromosome band 13q14; Yunis and Ramsay 1978) and the Wilms' tumour-aniridia, genitourinary abnormalities and mental retardation triad (WAGR; chromosome band 11p13; Riccardi et al. 1978, 1980; Francke et al. 1979). In both cases the deletions (loss of function) suggest the existence of tumour-suppressor genes within these regions. The retinoblastoma gene (Rb-1) has been cloned (Friend et al. 1986; Lee et al. 1987a) and its tumour-suppressor activity has been demonstrated (Huang et al. 1988). The gene encodes a protein with nuclear localization and DNA-binding capability (such as zinc-binding fingers) (Lee et al. 1987a,b) suggesting a regulatory function. Furthermore, in all retinoblastomas, both copies of the Rb gene are inactivated or transcribe altered mRNAs (Friend et al. 1986; Fung et al. 1987). The Rb gene product binds to several viral transforming proteins such as the E1A of the human adenovirus type 5, SV40 large T and human papilloma virus type 16 E7 oncogenes (summarized by Weinberg 1989), indicating that it might counteract these transforming proteins.

For the postulated Wilms' tumour gene at 11p13, a similar function might be expected. Evidence for suppressor activity on chromosome 11 comes from the experiments of Weismann et al. (1987), who demonstrated that the introduction of one normal chromosome 11 into a Wilms' tumour cell linne can supress malignancy. In addition, we demonstrated that fibroblast cell strains from patients with deletions of 11p13 are susceptible to morphological transformation

---

* This work has been supported by Netherlands Cancer Foundation (Koningin Wilhelmina Fonds) grant no IKA 89–30
[1] Institute of Human Genetics, University of Amsterdam, Academic Medical Centre, Meibergdreef 15, 1105 AZ Amsterdam ZO, The Netherlands
[2] The Netherlands Ophthalmic Research Institute, P.O. Box 12141, 1100 AC Amsterdam, The Netherlands
[3] Department of Biochemistry, Imperial College of Science and Technology, Imperial College Road, London SW7 2AZ, United Kingdom
[4] Emma Kinderziekenhuis/het kinder AMC, Academic Medical Centre, Meibergdreef 15, 1105 AZ Amsterdam ZO, The Netherlands
* *Present address*: Department of Genetics, Agricultural University, Dreyenlaan 2, 6703 HA Wageningen, The Netherlands

H.T. Lynch and P. Tautu (Eds.)
Recent Progress
in the Genetic Epidemiology of Cancer
© Springer-Verlag Berlin Heidelberg 1991

by early human polyomavirus BK DNA or to induction of anchorage-independent growth by human papillomavirus type 16 DNA, whereas normal diploid human fibroblasts are not (de Ronde et al. 1988; Smits et al. 1988). Chromosomal region 11p13 therefore may indeed contain a tumour-suppressor locus designated ST2 (HGM10 proceedings 1989). On the other hand, homozygous deletions of 11p13 in Wilms' tumour are very rare (1 reported case, Lewis et al. 1988) in contrast to retinoblastoma where deletions of 13q14 are frequently described as discussed before. Furthermore, the genetics of Wilms' tumour seems to be more complex than the genetics of retinoblastoma, as will be discussed later on.

Wilms' Tumour and Associated Congenital Diseases

Wilm's tumour is an embryonic nephroblastoma with an incidence of 1 per 10 000 children. It is usually diagnosed before the age of 7 years with a median age at diagnosis for unilateral unicentric tumours (86%) of 36.5 months for males and 42.5 months for females (Breslow et al. 1982, 1988). For bilateral cases (6%) these numbers are 23.5 and 30.5 months, respectively. The median age for multicentric unilateral cases (8%) is intermediate between the bilateral and unicentric medians. Several congenital diseases show an increased risk for Wilms' tumour, i.e., sporadic aniridia, the Beckwith-Wiedemann syndrome, hemihypertrophy, pseudohermaphroditism (Drash syndrome) and the Perlman and Klippel-Trenaunay syndromes. Of these, sporadic aniridia is most frequently associated with Wilms' tumour (33% of all cases), especially if it occurs together with various features of the AGR triad and a deletion in 11p13 (89% risk for Wilms' tumour; Moore et al. 1986). Patients with the Beckwith-Wiedemann syndrome have an overall tumour risk of 7.5%; 50% of these tumours are Wilms' tumours. The tumour risk is increased if hemihypertrophy is also present (40% in cases with Wilms' tumour compared with 12.5% in Beckwith-Wiedemann patients without Wilms' tumour). Other tumours frequently associated with the Beckwith-Wiedemann syndrome are rhabdomyosarcoma, hepatoblastoma and adreno-cortical carcinoma (Pettenati et al. 1986). A few patients with the Beckwith-Weidemann syndrome have been reported as having a duplication of 11p15.4-pter (Turleau and de Grouchy 1985), and the syndrome has been assigned to region 11p15 by linkage analysis (Koufos et al. 1989; Ping et al. 1989).

Wilms' tumour can occur in a sporadic or a familial form with a penetrance of 63% (Knudson and Strong 1972). On the basis of epidemiological investigations, Knudson and Strong (1972) proposed the "two-hit hypothesis" for the development of Wilms' tumour. They assumed that two mutations were required for the development of a Wilms' tumour, one of which could be inherited and would therefore be constitutional. Apart from the constitutional deletion of 11p13 in WAGR, abnormalities of 11p are also found in sporadic Wilms' tumours from individuals with an apparently normal constitutional karyotype (Kaneko et al. 1981; Slater and de Kraker 1972; Slater et al. 1985).

Loss of Heterozygosity in Wilms' Tumour

Recent studies on the loss of heterozygosity (LOH) have revealed the chromosomal localization of a number of genes whose inactivation or deletion is crucial
for the development of particular types of tumours (summarized by Ponder 1988).
In 1983, using molecular biological techniques, Cavenee et al. proposed that in
retinoblastoma recessive mutations can be revealed by chromosomal mechanisms such as unequal mitotic recombination, deletion, unbalanced translocations,
point mutations and aneuploid loss with endoreduplication. The first evidence
that this might be similar for chromosome 11p in Wilms' tumour came in 1984 from
several authors (Koufos et al. 1984; Eccles et al. 1984; Fearon et al. 1984; Reeve
et al. 1984; Orkin et al. 1984) who all found loss of heterozygosity of 11p15
markers. Some of these studies in human malignancies have also shown that a
number of different chromosomal regions associated with putative tumour
suppressor genes may be involved in any one given tumour. This was shown by
Vogelstein et al. 1989 who found that in colon carcinoma LOH involved a number
of different chromosomes and that increased LOH was associated with a poor
prognosis. Up until the present time no such data were available for Wilms'
tumour. Consequently, we have investigated LOH in a number of Wilms'
tumours using probes for regions containing most of the known proposed tumour
suppressor genes, namely probes for 3p, 5q, 11p, 13q, 17p and 22q (Mannens et
al. 1990). Examination of 44 tumours revealed LOH for 11p15 markers in 11 out
of 29 informative tumours (11 out of 36 informative tumours for 11p13 and 11p15
markers). Only one tumour had additional LOH involving probes for regions 5q
and 17p (Table 1). There was no correlation with tumour histology or stage of
development. No LOH for chromosome 11 markers was found in seven bilateral
cases. This lack of LOH (only one out of nine bilateral tumours showed loss of
chromosome 11 markers) has also been found by M. Little (personal communication). LOH was often present in stage I tumours as well, indicating that this
phenomenon is not a measure for the aggressiveness and metastatic properties of
the tumour. Moreover, the single tumour showing LOH on 5q, 11p and 17p was
also a stage I tumour. Thus our findings support a major role for chromosome 11p
in Wilms' tumour development and apparent non-involvement of other tumour
suppressor genes. An explanation for the finding that LOH in Wilms' tumour
seems to be restricted to chromosome 11, in contrast to the LOH for multiple
chromosomes found in adult tumours like breast and colon cancer, might be that

Table 1. Loss of heterozygosity (LOH) in Wilms' tumour (cases with LOH/number of informative cases)

N	3p	5q	11p	13q	17p	22q
44	0/16	1/17	11/29	0/17	1/27	0/19
	(N = 36)	(N = 31)	(N = 41)	(N = 34)	(N = 32)	(N = 33)

Markers tested: 3p (THR); 5q (D5S6); 11p (INS, HRAS1); 13q (RB1, D13S22); 17p (D17S5); 22q
(IGLV); N, number of cases investigated

Wilms' tumours are of embryonic origin. Thus the target cells are not fully differentiated and may need less mutational events to become tumorigenic than completely differentiated cells.

Chromosome Region 11P15

Using a range of probes for regions 11p15, 11p13 and 11q we were able to demonstrate that LOH occurred through the chromosomal mechanisms described earlier by Cavenee et al. (1983) for retinoblastoma (Mannens et al. 1988; Dao et al. 1987). We further noticed that in at least four out of 11 informative tumours showing LOH for chromosome 11, this LOH was limited to band 11p15.5 (Fig. 1). This finding was confirmed by others, demonstrating that LOH was

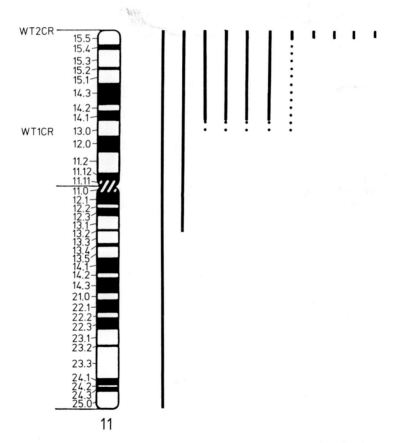

Fig. 1. Loss of heterozygosity on chromosome 11 in 44 Wilms' tumours. *Solid lines*: Regions showing LOH; *dotted lines*: markers not informative; *WT1CR*, Wilms' Tumour 1 chromosome region; *WT2CR*, Wilms' Tumour 2 chromosome region. Markers tested: 11p15 (HRAS1; INS); 11p13 (FSHB; D11S151; CAT); 11q (PGA; APOA1). In four cases, LOH for FSHB and/or D11S151 was found but CAT was not informative. Therefore it is unclear whether LOH occurred at the WT1 locus

limited to 11p15 in 50% of the informative tumours (Grundy et al. 1988; Koufos et al. 1989; Reeve et al. 1989). We and others found a highly significant preferential somatic loss of maternal alleles for this region in patients without a genetic predisposition to Wilms' tumour (Table 2). These data suggest that 11p15 is involved in Wilms' tumour development. Furthermore, in some WAGR patients with a constitutional deletion in 11p13 (Henry et al. 1989a) and in a familial case described by Grundy et al. (1988), the site for which an allele loss is observed in the tumour is 11p15 and not 11p13.

The preferential loss of maternal alleles in these embryonic tumours might reflect a relationship between tissue-specific imprinting (Sapienza 1989) and malignant growth as we have suggested previously (Mannens et al. 1988). Imprinting, involving a gamete of origin-dependent allele-inactivation process (Sapienza 1989), was also invoked to explain the maternal loss of alleles in rhabdomyosarcoma (Scrable et al. 1989), a tumour associated with the Beckwith-Wiedemann syndrome and 11p15 LOH, and osteosarcoma (Toguchida et al. 1989). Genomic imprinting has also been suggested as playing a role in hereditary glomus tumours (van der Mey et al. 1989), Prader-Willi syndrome (Nicholls et al. 1989), Huntington's chorea, Spinocerebellar ataxia, myotonic dystrophy and neurofibromatosis I and II (reviewed by Reik 1989) to explain the phenotypic variability in expression of these genetic disorders.

For the tumours described above, imprinting (for instance hyper- or hypomethylation of a gene) could have the same effect as a mutation at that locus. Such a gamete of origin-dependent imprint would last only for one generation. Therefore it could also explain why no linkage between predisposition for Wilms' tumour and 11p markers was observed in two large families (Huff et al. 1988; Grundy et al. 1988). It is an interesting speculation that the genetic predisposition for Wilms' tumour in these families is caused by a mutated gene that regulates imprinting of the 11p alleles associated with Wilms' tumour development.

Table 2. Loss of maternal alleles in patients without 2 genetic predisposition to Wilms' tumour

Reeve et al. 1984:	2/2
Schroeder et al. 1987:	3/3
Mannens et al. 1988:	3/3
Williams et al. 1989:	3/3
HGM10 and Washington chromosome 11 meeting, march 1989[a]:	5/5
Total	16/16

Only unilateral tumours from patients without 2 genetic predisposition to Wilms' tumour are listed. 16/16 tumours retained the paternal alleles ($p < 0.001 \; x^2$)

[a] Personal communication C Junien, C. Sapienza, G. Saunders, J. Cowell and co-workers

We have been able to demonstrate methylation differences for 11p markers between Wilms' tumour material and constitutional tissue of the patient (Mannens et al. 1988). However, it should be noted that this phenomenon is common to all tumour types or transformed cells investigated so far. For the Beckwith-Wiedemann syndrome, the imprinting model can also be applied since Aleck et al. (1989) reported an "ovum-mediated" transmission of the disease. We had the opportunity to investigate a nuclear family with a balanced translocation t(4,11) (p14;p15.5) found in mother and daughter. Although the mother had no clinical abnormalities, the child had all the characteristic features of the Beckwith-Wiedemann syndrome. Using the methylation-sensitive enzyme HpaII and its methylation-insensitive isoschizomere MspI, we could demonstrate that in the child the maternally derived allele of an RFLP marker in the insulin region (which is closely linked to the syndrome) was indeed hypomethylated compared with the same allele in the mother.

This suggests that the phenotypic effect of the de novo translocation was revealed after maternal transmission by demethylation. Cloning of the gene involved is necessary to confirm this finding.

Duplications of the 11p15 region in the Beckwith-Wiedemann syndrome have been described by several groups (see Turleau and de Grouchy 1985). Therefore we investigated a series of 15 nuclear Beckwith-Wiedemann families and we were unable to demonstrate any 11p15 abnormalities at the cytogenetic and DNA level. Apparently duplications occur only in a few cases. On the other

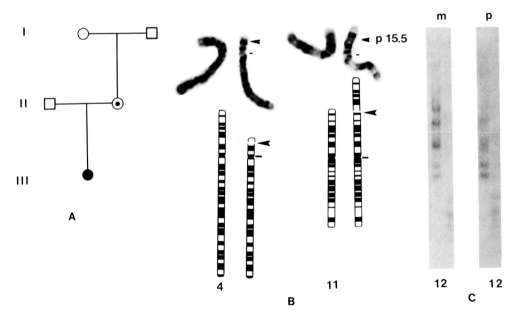

Fig. 2A-C. A family with a balanced t(4;11) (p14; *p15.5*) and a child with the Beckwith-Wiedemann syndrome. **A** Pedigree. Both mother and child carried the translocation. Only the child had the clinical features of the syndrome. **B** High-resolution banding of the translocation. **C** *Taq*I / *Hpa*II (*lanes* 1) and *Taq*I / *Msp*I (*lanes* 2) digests of mother (*m*) and child (*p*)

hand, by studying the two patients with 11p duplications, reported by Waziri et al. (1983), we were able to confirm their chromosome studies using DNA analysis and in situ hybridization.

The breakpoints in these patients occurred in 11p15 and 11p13, proximal to the CALCA gene and distal to the catalase gene, respectively. Henry et al. (1989b) described the smallest duplicated region in two patients being CALCA-pter, CALCA excluded.

Chromosome Region 11P13

For the 11p13 region there is no evidence for methylation variation as studied by pulsed field gel electrophoresis of CpG islands (Bickmore et al. 1989). Furthermore the homologous region in the mouse is not imprinted (reviewed by Reik 1989). On the other hand, Huff et al. (1989) reported paternal origin of de novo constitutional deletions in this region in seven out of eight aniridia patients. Five patients, including the patient with the deletion of maternal origin, developed a Wilms' tumour. Although this can be explained by an increased paternal mutation rate in the germline, this phenomenon could also reflect a more critical role for maternally derived genes in this region during early development.

Map of the 11P13 Region

Many breakpoints associated with Wilms' tumour, aniridia, genitourinary abnormalities (including a neonate with Potter's facies) and T-ALL have been mapped to the PFGE map of the WAGR region (summarized in the HGM10 proceedings 1989). The mapping of the Potter's translocation within 1 Mbp of the proposed Wilms' tumour locus (Porteous et al. 1987) suggests that renal dysplasia may be an alternative manifestation of mutation at the Wilms' tumour locus. Alternatively the Wilms' tumour gene may be part of a cluster of genes involved in genitourinary development (Bickmore et al. 1990). The aniridia gene has also been mapped to this region by linkage analysis of a large Dutch family with normal karyotype between the catalase ($\hat{z} = 7.27$ at $\hat{\theta} = 0.00$) and D11S151 ($\hat{z} = 3.86$ at $\hat{\theta} = 0.10$) markers (Mannens et al. 1989). Using flanking markers for this aniridia gene we were able to show that one member of this family with only nystagmus but no visible iris loss was, according to our findings, not a carrier for aniridia, although nystagmus is very often seen in aniridia patients and variability in expression for aniridia has been reported (Delleman and Winkelman 1973).

The genes for Wilms' tumour and aniridia are separated by several markers, including the D11S323 and D11S324 markers (gene order: CAT − D11S325 − S1 − Wilms' tumour − D11S323/D11S324 − aniridia − D11S16 − D11S151 (HGM10 proceedings 1989). These markers can therefore be used to identify the aniridia patients at risk for Wilms' tumour. Our molecular and cytogenetic analyses of a large series of patients with various features of the WAGR syndrome revealed that all of the 23 investigated patients having no deletions for these markers did not develop a Wilms' tumour. Two patients had not reached the age of 3 years (median age of risk) and are still at risk. Six patients had not reached the age of 7 years. In ten additional cases we detected deletions with all markers spanning the WAGR region. Three patients developed a Wilms' tumour; two additional patients are still at risk. Two patients had duplications of the WAGR region. Only one child was mildly mentally retarded. No other clinical abnormalities were found in these two patients. Surprisingly, we found no deletions with any of the above-mentioned markers in six bilateral Wilms' tumour patients (two with mental retardation and genitourinary abnormalities) and two aniridia patients with genitourinary abnormalities.

Two candidate sequences for the Wilms' tumour gene have been isolated (Call et al. 1989; Ton et al. 1989) that map within a 300 kb fragment of the postulated Wilms' tumour locus. Both cDNAs detect transcripts that are expressed predominantly in the kidney. Call et al. (1989) found that their DNA sequence codes for a protein with at least four zinc-binding fingers. Northern blot analysis revealed that this mRNA is absent or decreased in several Wilms' tumour cell lines. Recently, a series of cosmids with zinc-binding finger motifs have been isolated from a cosmid library derived from a human-mouse chromosome 11p enriched hybrid cell line (Porteous et al. 1989) at the department of Biochemistry of the Imperial College of Science and Technology in London. Using in situ hybridization techniques we have so far been able to map one of these cosmids to the distal region of 11p13 and an additional cosmid to 11p15 and others to chromosomes 3 and 19. These cosmids might also be valuable for the study of 11p regions involved in Wilms' tumour and associated congenital diseases.

Summary

At least three loci seem to be involved in Wilms' tumour development: one at 11p13, associated with aniridia-genitourinary abnormalities and mental retardation; one at 11p15, associated with the Beckwith-Wiedemann syndrome; and one additional locus predisposing for familial Wilms' tumour not linked to 11p13 and 11p15 markers. This complicates the application of the theory of Knudson and Strong (1972), explaining hereditary and sporadic forms of Wilms' tumour with a two-hit model. It still remains to be sorted out whether both alleles of a tumour-suppressor gene have to be inactivated or whether two or more hits at multiple loci are necessary for a Wilms' tumour to develop.

Characterization of the now-identified Wilms' tumour loci, and analysis of mutations in these loci in Wilms' tumour cells, will help us to solve these questions. Such an approach would also enable us to study tumour-suppressor activity, if any, of genes in the identified loci, and to analyse the contribution of genomic imprinting to the aetiology of Wilms' tumour.

References

Aleck KA, Hadro TA (1989) Dominant inheritance of Wiedemann-Beckwith syndrome. Am J Med Genet 33:155–160

Bickmore WA, Hastie ND (1989) Aniridia, Wilms' tumor and human chromosome 11. Ophthalmic Paediatr Genet vol 10, 4:229–248

Bickmore WA, Porteous DJ, Christie S, Seawright A, Fletcher JM, Maule JC, Couillin P, Junien C, Hastie ND, Heyningen V van (1989) CpG islands surround a DNA segment located between translocation breakpoints associated with genitourinary dysplasia and aniridia. Genomics 5:685–693

Breslow NE, Beckwith JB (1982) Epidemiological features of Wilms' tumor: results of the national Wilms' tumor study. JNCI 68 (3):429–436

Breslow NE, Beckwith JB, Ciol M, Sharples K (1988) Age distribution of Wilms' tumor: report from the national Wilms' tumor study. Cancer Res 48:1653–1657

Call KM, Ito C, Buckler A, Pelletier D, Haber D, Glaser T, Rose E, Jones C, Housman D (1989) Isolation of a cDNA in the WAGR region: a candidate gene for Wilms' tumor (abstract). Am J Hum Genet 45(4):A179

Cavenee WK, Dryja TP, Philips RA, Benedict WF, Godbout R, Gallie BL, Murphree AL, Strong LC, White RL (1983) Expression of recessive alleles by chromosomal mechanisms in retinoblastoma. Nature 305:779–784

Dao DD, Schroeder WT, Chao LY, Kikuchi H, Strong LC, Riccardi VM, Pathak S, Nichols WW, Lewis WH, Saunders GF (1987) Genetic mechanisms of tumor-specific loss of 11p DNA sequences in Wilms' tumor. Am J Hum Genet 41:202–217

Delleman JW, Winkelman JE (1973) Die bedeutung der atypischen Kolobome und Defekte der Iris fur die Erkennung des hereditaren Aniridia-Syndroms. Klin Monatsbl Augenheilkd 163:528–542

Eccles MR, Millow LJ, Wilkins RJ, Reeve AE (1984) Harvey-ras allele deletion detected by in situ hybridization to Wilms' tumor chromosomes. Hum Genet 67:190–192

Fearon ER, Vogelstein B, Feinberg AP (1984) Somatic deletion and duplication of genes on chromosome 11 in Wilms' tumours. Nature 309:176–178

Francke U, Holmes LB, Atkins L, Riccardi VM (1979) Aniridia-Wilms' tumor association: evidence for specific deletion of 11p13. Cytogenet Cell Genet 24:185–192

Friend SH, Bernards R, Rogelj S, Weinberg RA, Rapaport JM, Albert DM, Dryja TP (1986) A human DNA segment with properties of the gene that predisposes to retinoblastoma and osteosarcoma. Nature 323:643–646

Fung YKT, Murphree AL, T'Ang A, Qian J, Hinrichs SH, Benedict WF (1987) Structural evidence for the authenticity of the human retinoblastoma gene. Science 236:1657–1661

Grundy P, Koufos A, Morgan K, Li FP, Meadows AT, Cavenee WK (1988) Familial predisposition to Wilms' tumor does not map to the short arm of chromosome 11. Nature 336:374–378

Henry I, Grandjouan S, Couillin P, Barichard F, Huerre Jeanpierre C, Glaser T, Philip T, Lenoir G, Chaussain JL, Junien C (1989a) Tumor-specific loss of 11p15.5 alleles in del11p13 Wilms' tumor and in familial adrenocortical carcinoma. Proc Natl Acad Sci USA 86:3247–3251

Henry I, Jeanpierre M, Couillin P, Barichard F, Serre JL, Journel H, Lamoureaux A, Turleau C, de Grouchy J, Junien C (1989b) Molecular definition of the 11p15.5 region involved in Beckwith-Wiedemann syndrome and probably in predisposition to adrenocortical carcinoma. Hum Genet 81:273–277

Huang HJS, Yee JK, Shew JY, Chen PL, Bookstein R, Friedmann T, Lee EYHP, Lee WH (1988) Suppression of the neoplastic phenotype by replacement of the Rb gene in human cancer cells. Oncogene 3:345–348

Huff V, Compton DA, Chao LY, Strong LC, Geiser CF, Saunders GF (1988) Lack of linkage of familial Wilms' tumour to chromosomal band 11p13. Nature 336:377–378

Huff V, Compton DA, Chao LY, Riccardi VM, Strong LC, Saunders GF (1989) Parental origin of de novo constitutional deletions of chromosomal band 11p13 (abstract). Am J Hum Genet 45(4):A25

Human Gene Mapping 10 (1989) 10th international workshop on human gene mapping. Cytogenet Cell Genet 51:1–4

Kaneko Y, Euges MC, Rowley JD (1981) Interstitial deletion of short arm of chromosome 11 limited to Wilms' tumor cells in a patient without aniridia. Cancer Res 41:4577–4578

Knudson AG, Strong LC (1972) Mutation and cancer: a model for Wilms' tumour of the kidney. J Natl Cancer Inst 48:313–323

Koufos A, Hansen MF, Lampkin BC, Workman ML, Copeland NG, Jenkins NA, Cavenee WK (1984) Loss of alleles at loci on human chromosome 11 during genesis of Wilms' tumour. Nature 309:170–172

Koufos A, Grundy P, Morgan K, Aleck KA, Hadro T, Lampkin BC, Kalbakji A, Cavenee WK (1989) Familial Wiedemann-Beckwith syndrome and a second Wilms' tumor locus both map to 11p15.5. Am J Hum Genet 44:711–719

Lee WH, Bookstein R, Hong F, Young LJ, Shew Y, Lee EY (1987a) Human retinoblastoma susceptibility gene: cloning, identification, and sequence. Science 235:1394–1399

Lee WH, Shew JY, Hong FD, Sery TW, Donoso LA, Young LJ, Bookstein R, Lee EY (1987b) The retinoblastoma susceptibility gene encodes a nuclear phosphoprotein associated with DNA binding activity. Nature 329:642–647

Lewis WH, Yeger H, Bonetta L, Chan HSL, Kang J, Jumien C, Cowell J, Jones C, Dafoe LA (1988) Homozygous deletion of a DNA marker from chromosome 11p13 in sporadic Wilms' tumour. Genomics 3:25–31

Mannens M, Slater RM, Heyting C, Bliek J, de Kraker J, de Pagter-Holthuizen P, Pearson PL (1988) Molecular nature of genetic changes resulting in loss of heterozygosity of chromosome 11 in Wilms' tumours. Hum Genet 81:41–48

Mannens M, Bleeker-Wagemakers EM, Bliek J, Hoovers J, Mandjes I, Tol S van, Frants RR, Heyting C, Westerveld A, Slater RM (1989) Autosomal dominant aniridia linked to the chromosome 11p13 markers catalase and D11S151 in a large Dutch pedigree. Cytogenet Cell Genet 52:32–36

Mannens M, Devilee P, Bliek J, Mandjes I, de Kraker J, Heyting C, Slater RM, Westerveld A (1990) Loss of heterozygosity in Wilms' tumors, studied for six putative tumor-suppressor regions, is limited to chromosome 11. Cancer Research 50:3279–3283

Mey AGL van der, Maaswinkel-Mooy PD, Cornelisse CJ, Schmidt PH, Kamp JJP van de (1989) Genomic imprinting in hereditary glomus tumors: evidence for new genetic theory. Lancet II:1291–1294

Moore JW, Hyman S, Antonarakis SE, Mules EH, Thomas GH (1986) Familial isolated aniridia associated with a translocation involving chromosomes 11 and 22 [t(11;22) (p13;q12.2)]. Hum Genet 72:297–302

Nicholls RD, Knoll HM, Butler MG, Karam S, Lalande M (1989) Genetic imprinting suggested by maternal heterodisomy in nondeletion Prader-Willi syndrome. Nature 342:281–285

Orkin SH, Goldman DS, Sallan SE (1984) Development of homozygosity for chromosome 11p markers in Wilms' tumor. Nature 309:172–174

Pettenati MJ, Haines JL, Higgins RR, Wappner RS, Palmer CG, Weaver DD (1986) Wiedemann-Beckwith syndrome: presentation of clinical and cytogenetic data on 22 new cases and review of the literature. Hum Genet 74:143–154

Ping AJ, Reeve AE, Law DJ, Young MR, Boehnke M, Feinberg AP (1989) Genetic linkage of Beckwith-Wiedemann syndrome to 11p15. Am J Hum Genet 44:720–723

Ponder B (1988) Gene losses in human tumors. Nature 335:400–402

Porteous DJ, Bickmore W, Christie S, Boyd PA, Cranston G, Fletcher JM, Gosden JR, Rout D, Seawright A, Simola KOJ, Van Heyningen V, Hastie ND (1987) HRAS1-selected chromosome transfer generates markers that colocalize aniridia- and genitourinary dysplasia-associated translocation breakpoints and the Wilms' tumor gene within band 11p13. Proc Natl Acad Sci USA 84:5355–5359

Porteous DJ, Wilkinson MM, Fletcher JM, Heyningen V van (1989) Human-mouse hybrids carrying fragments of single human chromosomes selected by tumor growth. Genomics 5:680–684

Reeve AE, Housiaux PJ, Gardner RJM, Chewings WE, Grindley RM, Millow LJ (1984) Loss of a Harvey ras allele in sporadic Wilms' tumor. Nature 309:174–176

Reeve AE, Sih SA, Raizis AM, Feinberg AP (1989) Loss of allelic heterozygosity at a second locus on chromosome 11 in sporadic Wilms' tumor cells. Mol Cell Biol 9:1799–1803

Reik W (1989) Genomic imprinting and genetic disorders in man. Trends Genet 5(10):331–336

Riccardi VM, Sujanski E, Smith AC, Francke U (1978) Chromosomal imbalance in the aniridia-Wilms' tumor association: 11p interstitial deletion. Pediatrics 61:604–610

Riccardi VM, Hittner HM, Francke U, Yunis JJ, Ledbetter D, Borges W (1980) The aniridia-Wilms' tumor association: the critical role of chromosome band 11p13. Cancer Genet Cytogenet 2:131–137

Ronde A de, Mannens M, Slater RM, Hoovers J, Heyting C, Bleeker-Wagemakers EM, Leschot NJ, Strien A van, Sol CJA, Schegget J ter, der Noordaa J van (1988) Morphological transformation by early region human polyomavirus BK DNA of human fibroblasts with deletions in the short arm of one chromosome 11. J Gen Virol 69:467–471

Sapienza C, Tran TH, Paquette J, McGowan R, Peterson A (1989) A methylation model for mammalian genome imprinting. Prog Nucleic Acids Res Mol Biol:145–157

Schroeder WT, Chao LY, Dao DD, Strong LC, Pathak S, Riccardi V, Lewis WH, Saunders GF (1987). Nonrandom loss of maternal chromosome 11 alleles in Wilms' tumors. Am J Hum Genet 40:413–420

Scrable H, Cavenee W, Ghavimi F, Lovell M, Morgan K, Sapienza C (1989) A model for embryonal rhabdomyosarcoma tumorigenisis that involves imprinting. Proc Natl Acad Sci USA 86:7480–7484

Slater RM, Kraker J de (1982) Chromosome number 11 and Wilms' tumor. Cancer Genet Cytogenet 5:237–245

Slater RM, Kraker J de, Voute PA, Delemarre JFM (1985) A cytogenetic study of Wilms' tumor. Cancer Genet Cytogenet 14:95–109

Smits HL, Raadsheer E, Rood I, Mehendale S, Slater RM, Noordaa J van der, Schegget J ter (1988) Induction of anchorage-independent growth of human embryonic fibroblasts with a deletion in the short arm of chromosome 11 by human papillomavirus type 16 DNA. J Virol 62(12):4538–4543

Toguchida J, Ishizaki K, Sazaki MS, Nakamura Y, Ikenaga M, Kato M, Sugimoto M, Kotoura Y, Yamamuro T (1989) Preferential mutation of paternally derived RB gene as the initial event in sporadic osteosarcoma. Nature 338:156–158

Ton CCT, Weil MM, Compton DA, Tomlinson G, Miwa H, Strong LC, Saunders GF (1989) Search for transcription units in the vicinity of the putative Wilms' tumor locus (abstract). Am J Hum Genet 45(4):A225

Turleau C, de Grouchy J (1985) Beckwith-Wiedemann syndrome: clinical comparison between patients with and without 11p15 trisomy. Ann Genet (Paris) 28:93–96

Vogelstein B, Fearon ER, Kern SE, Hamilton SR, Preisinger AC, Nakamura Y, White R (1989) Allelotype of colorectal carcinomas. Science 244:207–211

Waziri M, Shivanand RP, Hanson JW, Bartley JA (1983) Abnormality of chromosome 11 in patients with features of Beckwith-Wiedemann syndrome. J Pediatr 102:873–876

Weinberg RA (1989) Oncogenes, antioncogenes, and the molecular bases of multistep carcinogenisis. Cancer Res 49:3713–3721

Weismann BE, Saxon PJ, Pasquale SR, Jones GR, Geiser AG, Stanbridge EJ (1987) Introduction of a normal human chromosome 11 into a Wilms' tumor cell line controls its tumorigenic expression. Science 236:175–236

Williams JC, Brown KW, Mott MG, Maitland NJ (1989) Maternal allele loss in Wilms' tumor. Lancet 1:283–284

Yunis JJ, Ramsey N (1978) Retinoblastoma and subband deletion of chromosome 13. Am J Dis Child 132:161–163

Analysis of Association in Nuclear Families*

S.A. Seuchter[1], M. Knapp, and M.P. Baur

Introduction

The major goal of association studies in genetics is to define risk haplotypes which may be responsible for the disease phenotype and to determine what kind of genetic control the marker system contributes to the disease, which may help then in better understanding the mode of inheritance for complex diseases.

There can be several causes for phenotypic associations and one should be aware of them when studying associations. Phenotypic association may be due to sampling from a heterogeneous population, e.g., a population containing a subpopulation where a specific antigen and the disease are in a lower or higher frequency (Ott 1988). Additionally, tight linkage (the recombination fraction is small) maintains association caused by selection, mixing of population, random fluctuation and other population forces, whereas without linkage (the recombination fraction equals ½) these associations decay rapidly over generations (Thompson 1986). Thus, the observation of the same association throughout several generations may be indicative for linkage, but does not prove it. Another cause for phenotypic association is epistasis. This is the interaction of the phenotypic expression between alleles of different loci which need not necessarily be linked (Morton 1982). Furthermore gene-environment interaction may also be the reason for an association. However, studies concerned with gene-environment interaction have been mainly limited to drug sensitivity and major locus genotypes, e.g., the antimalarial drug primaquine induces hemolytic anemia in men only with a particular allele at a sex-linked locus. The greatest challenge in genetic epidemiology is probably to determine gene-environmental interaction. Clearly, genetic models are best determined by the use of data from related individuals and environmental components are best determined by the use of case-control or cohort data. The only way of appropriately merging these two fields seems to be to first map a gene and then study a cohort of individuals with the susceptible genotype and a set of controls, so that gene-environmental interaction can be defined (Skolnick 1987).

* This work was supported by BMFT project 01ZU8804/0 and DFG Ba 660/5–3

[1] Institute for Medical Statistics, Sigmund-Freud Straße 25, W-5300 Bonn 1, FRG

H.T. Lynch and P. Tautu (Eds.)
Recent Progress
in the Genetic Epidemiology of Cancer
© Springer-Verlag Berlin Heidelberg 1991

Materials and Methods

The Relative Risk

The strength of association is measured by the relative risk (RR), which is defined as the probability ratio of contracting a disease, given that a certain trait or condition is present, over that of the population. The odds ratio as proposed by Woolf is a good approximation of the true RR if the overall prevalence of the disease in the population is low (Woolf 1955).

The RR has also been applied in genetics to estimate risks for genetic markers associated with many diseases. Its most notable use has been in studying HLA-associated diseases (Thomson 1981). To be applied in genetics however, several assumptions about the underlying population have to be made, most importantly the disease and control sample should originate from the same genetically homogenous background. In practice this is rather difficult to fulfill.

The Haplotype Relative Risk

As an alternative risk measurement the haplotype relative risk (HRR) was proposed by Rubinstein et al. 1981. This constructs its own internal control sample from those parental haplotypes not transmitted to the affected child. However, it requires other important conditions which are outlined by Falk and Rubinstein (1987) and Ott (1988).

In practice, these conditions can rarely be completely satisfied, as for example in our systematic lupus erythematosus (SLE) family study. SLE is an autoimmune disease which is thought to be associated with alleles of the HLA complex, like many other diseases. The HLA complex consists of highly polymorphic loci which control the cell surface antigens and provoke intense immunologic response when foreign antigens are recognized. Our study includes families ascertained through one affected individual (not necessarily an affected child) and marker information from several family members with partially missing data.

The Haplotype Frequency Difference (HFD)

Model

Consider a multiallelic marker locus, e.g., the HLA complex (a codominant system with one recessive allele), with the alleles $a_0,...,a_n$. The genetic model of the disease phenotype assumes a diallelic disease locus where n denotes the disease-predisposing allele, N the normal allele, and p is the population frequency of n. Then, the frequency of allele a_i among the affected haplotypes is defined as:

$$v_i = \frac{P(a_i\ n)}{p} \tag{1}$$

the conditional probability of allele a_i at the marker locus given the allele n at the disease locus. The population frequency of the marker allele a_i is represented by q_i. Assuming a recessive mode of inheritance with incomplete penetrance, both haplotypes of the proband must carry the disease-predisposing allele and therefore v_i equals the frequency of allele a_i under the transmitted parental haplotypes, and the frequency for the non-transmitted haplotypes is equal to the population probability q_i of the marker allele a_i. Thus, this sample of non-transmitted haplotypes represents a random sample of the general population. In case of no association between the disease and marker allele a_i, the haplotype frequency difference

$$\text{Dif}_i := v_i - q_i \tag{2}$$

equals zero.

Estimation

Estimation of the haplotype frequency difference between the transmitted and nontransmitted haplotypes requires estimation of v_i and q_i, which we do by calculating the maximum likelihood estimators (MLE) $\hat{v}_i$ and $\hat{q}_i$. These MLEs are obtained by the family analysis package FAP (Neugebauer et al. 1984; Seuchter et al. 1990).

Statistical Inference

Besides estimating the haplotype frequency difference between the transmitted and nontransmitted haplotypes, usually one is interested in testing departures of this difference from zero. Hence, a decision between the hypotheses

$$H_0 : \text{Dif}_i = 0 \quad \text{vs} \quad H_1 : \text{Dif}_i \neq 0 \tag{3}$$

has to be determined. The estimated haplotype frequency difference $\widehat{\text{Dif}}$ (we suppress the index i from now on) is asymptotically normal distributed with expectation zero under the null hypothesis. Of course, the exact variance of the estimated difference is not known. To circumvent this problem we use the leaving-one-out or Jackknife estimator (Efron 1982) for the variance which is defined as

$$\widehat{\text{Var}(\widehat{\text{Dif}})} = \frac{m-1}{m} \sum_{j=1}^{m} (\widehat{\text{Dif}_{(j)}} - \overline{\text{Dif}_{(.)}})^2 \tag{4}$$

where

$$\overline{\text{Dif}_{(.)}} = \frac{1}{m} \sum_{j=1}^{m} (\widehat{\text{Dif}_{(j)}}) \tag{5}$$

(m denotes the total number of families)

and $\widehat{\text{Dif}_{(j)}}$ in (4) denotes the MLE for the haplotype frequency difference based on the sample without the jth family. Then an appropriate test statistic is

$$\text{HFD:} = \frac{\text{Dif}}{\sqrt{\text{Var}(\widehat{\text{Dif}})}} \tag{6}$$

the haplotype frequency difference between the transmitted and nontransmitted a_i marker allele over all m families divided by the standard deviation of the haplotype frequency difference. Under the null hypothesis, the HFD is asymptotically standard normal distributed.

The value of the HFD has to be compared with the $1-\alpha/2$ quantile of the standard normal distribution.

Application

Using the collected 132 SLE families from the multicenter study with caucasian background (Hartung et al. 1989) we applied the HFD statistic to the HLA DR locus. Table 1 shows the results obtained for the DR alleles. As seen in this table, the null hypothesis of no deviation of the haplotype frequency difference between the transmitted v_i and the nontransmitted q_i from zero could be firmly rejected for the DR1, DR2, DR3 and DR5 alleles, where for the DR2 and DR3 alleles a higher frequency has been observed for the transmitted, and for the DR1 and DR5 alleles a higher frequency in the nontransmitted haplotypes has been identified. DR1 and DR5 alleles may have a protective effect for the disease phenotype. However, another reason for this low frequency in the transmitted DR1 and DR5 haplotypes is also that if one allele has a higher frequency consequently the frequency of another allele has to be lower.

Table 1. Analysis of the haplotype frequency difference (HFD) statistic applied to the DR locus

Allele	$\hat{v}_i$	$\hat{q}_i$	$\widehat{\text{Dif}}_i$	$\widehat{\text{Var}(\text{Dif})}$	HFD	p-value[a]
DR1	0.0510	0.1467	−0.096	0.0008	−3.3205	0.0009
DR2	0.2367	0.1304	0.107	0.0423	2.5967	0.0094
DR3	0.2842	0.1076	0.177	0.0062	4.6961	<0.0001
DR4	0.0882	0.1330	−0.045	0.0499	−1.4301	0.1527
DR5	0.0807	0.1712	−0.091	0.0035	−2.3965	0.0166
DR6	0.0957	0.1512	−0.055	0.0028	−1.4260	0.1539
DR7	0.0924	0.1076	−0.015	0.0024	−0.5037	0.6145
DR8	0.0159	0.0243	−0.009	0.0003	−0.5382	0.5904
DR9	0.0040	0.0095	−0.006	0.0001	−0.5602	0.5753
DR0	0.0511	0.0089	0.042	0.0036	1.3732	0.1697

$\hat{v}_i$ = estimated frequency of allele a_i among haplotypes transmitted to the affected individuals.
$\hat{q}_i$ = estimated frequency of allele a_i among haplotypes *not* transmitted to the affected individuals.
[a] p-value based on the standard normal distribution.

Discussion

The discovery of associations of specific histocompatibility (HLA) antigens with several diseases (hemochromatosis, ankylosing spondylitis, etc.) offers promise of resolving the mode of inheritance of the disease. If a high association has been reported between a disease and a specific antigen, one could suggest that this association is due to tight linkage between the HLA loci and the loci which control susceptibility to those diseases. However, these associations have to be confirmed by independent studies so that one can exclude the effects of population structures.

The problem in studying associations is to ensure that both samples originate from the same homogeneous population, which in practice is rather difficult to fulfill. Additionally, analyzing a marker system with one recessive allele, as for example the HLA system, introduces the problem of nondirectly observable alleles. Knapp et al. (submitted) show that the effect of including only unique family patterns for the analysis will result in a selection bias. They have investigated several strategies for estimating and testing the HRR for marker systems with one recessive allele. One of them, the haplotype frequency difference statistic, has been applied to the DR locus of 132 families of our SLE study. In this study, families have been ascertained through one affected individual and not necessarily an affected child, since this disease has a rather late age of onset. The advantage of using the MLE for transmitted and nontransmitted haplotype frequency differences is that in the estimation process all family patterns are regarded including those with incomplete genotype information. The assumption of a recessive mode of inheritance is actually a conservative approach, since if for example in reality a dominant mode of inheritance would be the true one, a bias will be introduced in the estimation of v_i towards q_i, resulting in a smaller haplotype frequency difference.

Further investigations of the association between diseases and marker systems with one recessive allele will focus on methods for risk calculations of extended haplotypes and on the risks for particular genotypes. Although these methods presented here have been used for autoimmune diseases, their application is also valid for any other disease (breast cancer, melanoma, etc.).

References

Efron B (1982) The Jackknife, the Bootstrap and other resampling plans. Society for Industrial and Applied Mathematics, Philadelphia

Falk C, Rubinstein P (1987) Haplotype relative risk: an easy reliable way to construct a proper control sample for risk calculation. Ann Hum Genet 51:227–233

Hartung K, Riedel T, Stannat S, Specker C, Röther E, Pirner K, Schendel D, Baur M, Schneider P, Rittner C, Peter HH, Lakomek HJ, Kalden JR, Deicher H (1989) The association of major histocompatibility complex loci with systematic lupus erythematosus — role of C4Q0-Alleles (Abstract). 7th International Congress of Immunology, Berlin

Morton NE (1982) Association. In: Morton NE et al. (eds) Outline of genetic epidemiology. Karger, Basel, pp 89–104

Neugebauer M, Willems J, Baur MP (1984) Analysis of multilocus pedigree data by computer. In: Albert ED, Baur MP, Mayr WR (eds) Histocompatibility testing 1984. Springer, Berlin Heidelberg New York, pp 52–58

Ott J (1985) Association between phenotypes at two loci. In: Ott J et al. (eds) Analysis of human genetic linkage. Johns Hopkins University Press. Baltimore, pp 147–165

Ott J (1989) Statistical properties of the haplotype relative risk. Genet Epidemiol 6:127–130

Rubinstein P, Walker M, Carpenter C, Carrier C, Krassner C, Ginsberg F (1981) Genetics of HLA disease associations. The use of the haplotype relative risk (HRR) and the "haplo-delta" (Dh) estimates in juvenile diabetes from three racial groups. Hum Immunol 3:384

Seuchter SA, Neugebauer M, Baur MP (1990) Usermanual for FAP — Family Analysis Package. Institute for Medical Statistics, University of Bonn, West Germany

Skolnick MH (1987) Priority needs in the development of genetic epidemiology. In: Draggon S, Cohrssen JJ, Morrison RE (eds) Environmental impacts on human health. Praeger, London, pp 15–33

Thompson EA (1986) A brief introduction of human genetics. In: Thompson EA et al. (eds) Pedigree analysis in human genetics. John Hopkins Press, Baltimore, pp 1–15

Thomson G (1981) A review of theoretical aspects of HLA and disease associations. Theor Popul Biol 20/2:168–208

Woolf B (1955) On estimating the relation between blood group and disease. Ann Hum Genet 19:251–253

Ascertainment Problems in Family Data: Methodological Aspects

J. STENE

Introduction

Family data are commonly used in many fields of medicine and social sciences. A family consists of a group of individuals sharing a number of biological and social relations. The definition of a family may vary with the actual context. It may denote a biological, nuclear family consisting of biological children of the same two parents. The term may also include more complex groups where the females may have had children with different males and the males children with different females. Often the term may refer to a pedigree over more than two generations. In social sciences the term "family" may denote a household, whose members are not necessarily related.

One often finds that the type of family data used in a study has not been defined precisely. Several types may be used in the same study, e.g. both nuclear families and pedigrees are often used without any distinction being made between them.

As the members of a family are interrelated in many ways, they cannot be considered to be independently selected. Collection of data about different family members may take place in several stages. One typical example is the following:

(1) The original detection of one or more family members possessing the particular character of interest for the study;
(2) tracing and studying their parents;
(3) tracing other offspring of one or both parents and determining whether they have the actual character or not;
(4) tracing and studying other relatives of the parents.

The selection procedures applied in each of these stages will be different and have to be taken into account in the statistical models and methods used to analyse the data. Application of such selection procedures is often called "ascertainment of family data" and the methodological problems which arise are referred to as "ascertainment problems" or "corrections for ascertainment".

The purpose of the present paper is to discuss the particular use of the term "ascertainment", and address a few of the methodological problems, their effects on the conclusions if they are improperly dealt with and how they may be solved.

Institute of Statistics, University of Copenhagen, Studiestræde 6, 1455 Copenhagen K., Denmark

H.T. Lynch and P. Tautu (Eds.)
Recent Progress
in the Genetic Epidemiology of Cancer
© Springer-Verlag Berlin Heidelberg 1991

Reasons for Collecting Family Data

Family data may be collected in order to study the occurrence of some character within families characterized in a particular way, e.g. the family are living in a specified area or under certain specified conditions. One may have a hypothesis that the specified living conditions determine or at least have some influence on the occurrence frequency of the character, and that this frequency will vary with the conditions.

A different reason for collecting family data is to study the mode of inheritance of certain traits, e.g. inherited diseases. Many such traits are recessive and may be manifest among members of the offspring in a nuclear family but not in the parents. However, the parents will share between them a hidden genetic constitution that will cause them to have abnormal children of the observed type. The abnormality may be present at birth or appear later in life.

In purely genetical situations the frequency of the abnormal trait in the offspring is determined by the mode of inheritance only, which may be well defined in some cases.

More often, however, the frequencies are determined by both genetical and environmental factors, none of which are well defined, but the common environment of family members and their biological relationships make the use of family data an important tool for studies of such characters.

The Meaning of "Ascertainment of a Family"

As the use of the word "ascertainment" in the present context is somewhat imprecise, we will start by tracing its origin.

In order to simplify matters, we will confine ourselves mainly to the purely genetical situation. Consider a nuclear family with two apparently normal parents and s children, where r of these possess the recessive trait albinism, with $0 < r < s$ such that both normal and albino children are present. On the basis of these observations we infer that both parents are heterozygotes for the recessive gene for albinism.

If we want to study the mode of inheritance of albinism, or more precisely estimate the probability for a newborn child to be albino when both parents are heterozygotes, we collect a sample of nuclear families by the above-mentioned procedure starting with information about the offspring. Families where both parents are heterozygotes for this gene but by chance have no albino children will not be included in our sample. Thus our sample will be biased and, if we do not take this bias into account in our statistical model and methods, we will draw incorrect conclusions.

Here we have ascertained the genetic constitutions and mating types of the parents on the basis of observations on their children. The English verb "to ascertain" has been used for the last 150 years to mean: "to find out or learn for a certainty, to make sure of, get to know" (Little et al. 1973). These meanings are different from those of the verbs "to sample" and "to select", the common words used for collecting statistical data. The words "to ascertain" and "ascertainment" were first used in the present context by Fisher (1934). They were evidently translations from the German verb *erfassen* and the noun *Erfassung*, which had been introduced in this context by the German physician Weinberg more than 20 years earlier. Weinberg (1913) discusses at length the importance of determining the genetic constitutions of the parents and their mating type on the basis of observations on their offspring. He uses precisely the words *erfassen* and *Erfassung* for this way of drawing conclusions.

For the above-mentioned, biased sample of families, we have selected it by ascertaining the genetical constitutions of the parents and their mating type for each family. The so-called ascertainment bias arises here because we are unable to make such ascertainment without access to albino children.

Ascertainment bias will also arise if the probability for the ascertainment of the genetic constitution of the parents and their mating type increases with the number of abnormal children in the offspring.

It should be mentioned that a substantial part of the material in the above-mentioned paper by Fisher (1934) was, in fact, borrowed from earlier papers by Weinberg, even though Weinberg was neither cited nor mentioned by name. Extensive claims in the Anglo-American literature citing Fisher as the founder of this work are, therefore, not warranted.

The word "ascertainment" is frequently used in a looser sense when one has a hypothesis that the disposition for a disorder, e.g. a type of cancer, may be genetically determined, perhaps through several genes, but that the actual manifestation may be caused by additional factors. Also in this case the family data are collected on the basis of observed, abnormal offspring, in order to study the mode of inheritance of the disorder. However, to determine the genetic constitutions of the parents and their mating type, as far as the actual genes are concerned, may be very difficult.

In recent years the word "ascertainment" has increasingly been used more or less synonymously with "data selection" or "data sampling" in some medical contexts. In these cases observations are made on individuals or fetuses, but no conclusions are drawn about hidden properties in the parents. This abuse of the word should be avoided.

Sampling of Family Data

Family data of this kind could, in principle, be sampled by a two-stage procedure where the first stage consists of families selected by one of the standard methods of survey sampling, e.g. simple random sampling. In the second stage the sample may be selected by means of the ascertainment procedure mentioned above, by including only those families which had at least one albino child (or with the actual recessive trait). If a family has at least one albino child, the probability of the family being included in the sample would be independent of any additional albino children.

If the probability for a child in such a family to be albino is θ, then the conditional probability for a nuclear family with s children to have r albino children, given that it has been selected by means of this procedure, will be (with $1 \leq r \leq s$)

$$\binom{s}{r} \theta^r (1 - \theta)^{s-r} / [1 - (1 - \theta)^s] \tag{1}$$

This model is often called the complete ascertainment model and was suggested by Weinberg (1912a). In statistics it is known as truncated binomial distribution. Many estimation methods are available (Thomas and Gart 1971).

However, very few traits with such a simple mode of inheritance are so common that our data set, the second-stage sample (even with a very large, first-stage sample), would be sufficiently large to produce reasonably accurate estimates. An exception is seen in the common blood groups, e.g. the ABO system.

The usual situation is that a family is included in our data set simply on the basis of reports about one or more abnormal children. The initial, abnormal children (one or more in a family) who lead to the detection of the family are called probands (or index cases or propositi). In most cases no initial, formal, sampling procedure is applied in order to detect the probands.

For family data collected in this way the probability of a family being included in our data set may depend on the number of abnormal children, often in a complicated way, but also on a number of other family-related factors such as socio-economic status and location of family home.

Models for Family Data

In the last 30 years such family data have almost without exception been analysed by means of one single model for the data selection procedure, the so-called incomplete, multiple ascertainment model. In the simplified situation we considered, with a probability θ of a child being abnormal and the number of abnormals in the sibship being binomially distributed, the assumptions for this model are the following for each nuclear family:

(1) The family is found through individual probands, not pairs or groups of probands.
(2) The probands are detected independently of each other.
(3) The probability π for an abnormal child to be proband (often called the ascertainment probability for an abnormal) is the same for all abnormals in the family.
(4) The ascertainment probability is the same for all families with the actual type of abnormal offspring.

From these assumptions, the conditional probability that a family in our sample has r affected children and c independently selected probands, given that it has

s children and has been selected by means of the described procedure, will be (with $1 \leq c \leq r \leq s$)

$$f(r,c \mid s,\theta,\pi) = \frac{\binom{r}{c} \pi^c (1 - \pi)^{r-c} \binom{s}{r} \theta^r (1 - \theta)^{s-r}}{1 - (1 - \theta\pi)^s} \tag{2}$$

It should be stressed that when using this model one will automatically invoke these assumptions.

This model was introduced in this field by Weinberg (1912a,b) on the basis of his experiences in a related field. In Stuttgart, where he lived, he had access to the register of death certificates and to a register on families (Weinberg 1907). He could find cases where, for example, cancer or tuberculosis was given as the cause of death and then, in the family register, he could trace the families of these probands and find out if other sibs had died of the same cause or suffered from that disease. By this data-selection procedure the probability for an individual who had died of tuberculosis to be a proband was almost constant, and the assumption of independent probands could be considered to be approximately satisfied. For data selected in this or a similar way, the model is reasonable.

Except for a data-selection procedure such as that mentioned above, the model has very strong assumptions which are likely to be violated in real data. Only deviations from assumption 4 have been extensively discussed in the literature (see Stene 1981). We shall consider a couple of common deviations from the other assumptions and their consequences.

Varying Ascertainment Probability

The second and third assumptions for the model demand that the probands are detected independently and that the probability for an abnormal individual be the same for all abnormal sibs. If the family is reported as soon as one sib has manifested an abnormality, either at birth or later in life, the first affected sib will have a much higher probability of being a proband than any of the other abnormals. And as soon as the family has been included in the records of a hospital, where other cases of the same type may occur, it will be monitored such that additional cases will be recorded as a consequence of the monitoring, not as independently reported cases. Hence there will be only a single proband in each such family in our data set.

This reporting and monitoring pattern, which is common for a large number of severe and well-known abnormalities considered at least to be influenced by inherited factors, seriously contradicts assumptions 2 and 3.

It has been shown by Stene (1978) that the correct model for this data set is model 1, as the probability of the family being included in our data is independent of the number of abnormals (if there is at least one). However, had we used a computer program based on the incomplete, multiple ascertainment model 2, the ascertainment probability π would have been estimated as very small, and the recommended model would have been the so-called single ascertainment model with $1 \le r \le s$

$$\binom{s-1}{r-1} \theta^{r-1}(1-\theta)^{s-r} \tag{3}$$

If we had relied on the recommendations from the computer program, we would have chosen an incorrect model for our data, and the result would have been a serious underestimation of the segregation parameter θ, in particular if the families were small. The bias is independent of the number of families. The bias obtained by estimating θ on the basis of model 3 instead of 1 is illustrated in Table 1.

Table 1. Bias of estimate of θ by using model 3 instead of 1 for sibship sizes ($s = 2, 3, 5$ and 8)

	Bias (θ)			
s	0.1	0.3	0.5	0.7
2	−0.047	−0.123	−0.167	−0.161
3	−0.046	−0.115	−0.143	−0.121
5	−0.045	−0.099	−0.105	−0.073
8	−0.042	−0.079	−0.069	−0.042

Stene (1978) has shown that model 3 is a reasonable model for data sets of rare abnormalities which are neither well known nor severe, with only a single proband in each family, and where all abnormals have about the same probability of being the proband.

Simultaneous Reporting of More Abnormals

If an abnormality is relatively unknown, families are often reported if two or more sibs possess it. It may then be suspected that inheritance plays a role. In this case a pair or trio of probands will be simultaneously reported, not as independent probands as demanded by model 2. Alternative models for this type of ascertainment have been developed by Stene (1979).

Concluding Remarks

In this short paper only a few of the methodological problems in connection with the ascertainment of families have been touched. However, they should indicate that a thorough analysis of the ascertainment and selection problems involved are necessary in order to construct an appropriate model. An inappropriate model may lead to erroneous results.

References

Fisher RA (1934) The effect of methods of ascertainment upon the estimation of frequencies. Ann Eug 6:13–25

Little W, Fowler HW, Coulson Y, Onions CT (1973) The shorter Oxford English dictionary on historical principles, vol I. Clarendon, Oxford, p 112

Stene J (1978) Choice of ascertainment model I: discrimination between single-proband models by means of birth order data. Ann Hum Genet 42:219–229

Stene J (1979) Choice of ascertainment model II: discrimination between multi-proband models by means of birth order data. Ann Hum Genet 42:493–505

Stene J (1981) Probability distributions arising from the ascertainment and analysis of data on human families and other groups. In: Taillie C, Patil GP, Baldessari BA (eds) Statistical distributions in scientific work, vol 6. Reidel, Dortrecht, pp 233–264

Thomas DG, Gart JJ (1971) Small sample performance of some estimators of the truncated binomial distribution. J Am Stat Ass 66:169–177

Weinberg W (1907) Die württembergische Familienregister und ihre Bedeutung als Quelle wissenschaftlicher Untersuchungen. Württemb Jahrb Stat u Landeskunde 1907:174–198

Weinberg W (1912a) Über Methoden und Fehlerquellen der Untersuchung auf Mendelsche Zahlen beim Menschen. Arch Rassen Gesellsch Biol 9:165–174

Weinberg W (1912b) Zur Vererbung der Bluterkrankheit mit methodologischen Ergänzungen meiner Geschwistermethode. Arch Rassen Gesellsch Biol 9:694–709

Weinberg W (1913) Auslesewirkungen bei biologisch-statistischen Problemen I. Arch Rassen Gesellsch Biol 10:417–451

Polygenic vs Monogenic Inheritance of Dysplastic Nevi and Malignant Melanoma: Yesterday's Debate or the Answer of Tomorrow?

Heiko Traupe*

Introduction

The nature of genetic predisposition for malignant melanoma and dysplastic nevi is much debated. While the prevailing opinion today is that up to 10% of all melanomas are due to a mutation affecting a single gene (Bergman et al. 1986; Bale et al. 1986) we have questioned this view and have advanced a polygenic concept instead (Happle and Traupe 1982; Happle 1989; Traupe et al. 1989).

To some colleagues in human genetics and genetic epidemiology this may seem to be yesterday's debate. The concept of polygenic gene interaction has lost much of its shining glamour, mainly because it cannot be adequately tested with the currently available mathematical tools. As a consequence, it appears as a "black box" and tends to hide rather than to disclose the genes involved. Of course, the polygenes must also have a material substrate at the DNA level. Using recombinant DNA techniques many research groups currently try to isolate such specific genes in diseases previously thought to be polygenic. In some of these diseases spectacular advances have been achieved, for example in schizophrenia where a major gene could be assigned to chromosome 5 (Sherrington et al. 1988) or in colorectal carcinomas, where a loss of a tumor repressor gene borne on chromosome 5 has been demonstrated (Solomon et al. 1987).

The isolation of major predisposing genes in disorders thought to have a polygenic nature naturally has consequences on the polygenic concept and actually disproves an assumption often made for some of these diseases, namely that all genes contribute in a similar and equal manner. Some colleagues therefore now feel that the polygenic disease concept is more or less worthless and can be discarded. For them, the argument that dysplastic nevi and malignant melanomas are caused either by a single gene or by the additive action of major and minor genes may indeed appear to be yesterday's debate.

However, reviewing the available genetic and epidemiologic evidence, I shall conclude that this is not the case for malignant melanoma and that several genes are involved in the etiology of this tumor and its precursor lesions. Finally, I shall propose to test a three-major-gene concept which may well be the answer of tomorrow.

* The author is supported by the Deutsche Forschungsgemeinschaft (Grant Tr 228/1–2)

Department of Human Genetics, University of Nijmegen, P.O. Box 9101, 6500 HB Nijmegen, The Netherlands

H.T. Lynch and P. Tautu (Eds.)
Recent Progress
in the Genetic Epidemiology of Cancer
© Springer-Verlag Berlin Heidelberg 1991

The Historical Evolution of the Dysplastic Nevus Syndrome

Familial occurrence of malignant melanoma was first noted by Cawley (1952). He reported the disease in a father, daughter and son. In the ensuing years a number of similar case reports followed (Miller and Pack 1962; Salamon et al. 1963). In the early 1970s, two systematic studies established the existence of a hereditary predisposition to malignant melanoma (Anderson 1971; Wallace et al. 1971). Walace et al. (1971) investigated 125 newly diagnosed melanoma cases. Their study formed part of the Queensland melanoma project and they succeeded in gathering histories in 113 of their families, covering a total of 923 first degree relatives. Among these first degree relatives they observed 11 further cases of melanoma (incidence = 1.19%) instead of the expected 6.6 cases (based on an average incidence of 0.72% for melanoma in the general population of this area at that time). They concluded that 11% of their patients belonged to a melanoma family.

From the investigations by Anderson and Wallace a number of characteristic biologic features of familial melanoma emerged: taken as a group, familial melanomas are characterized by

(a) an early onset, usually before the age of 40 years,
(b) multiple occurrence,
(c) a much better overall prognosis,
(d) association with a fair complexion (with blond and red hair overrepresented), and
(e) association with multiple nevus cell nevi.

In 1978 Lynch et al. and Clark et al. independently reported on the association of familial melanomas with atypical moles and identified these moles as precursors of later evolving melanomas. Clinical and histologic criteria (Table 1) were

Table 1. Major clinical and histologic criteria for dysplastic nevi

Clinical features
Diameter of 5–12 mm
Macular and papular components
Irregular and ill-defined borders
Wide range in color from tan to dark-brown on a pink background
Occurrence also in covered areas

Histologic features
Basilar melanocytic hyperplasia with elongation of rete ridges
Cytologic atypia
Nest formation of melanocytes and fusing with adjacent rete ridges
Lamellar and concentric dermal fibroplasia
Inflammatory dermal infiltrates

None of these features is specific. Diagnosis relies on a combination of them

elaborated, separating these nevi from ordinary nevus cell nevi and characterizing them as potential precancerous lesions.

However, it soon became obvious that these atypical moles, (Fig. 1) which are now called "dysplastic nevi," not only occur in patients with familial melanomas but are also present in 30%–50% of patients with sporadic melanomas and in 2%–10% of the general population in individuals without a family history of melanoma (Tucker 1988; Steijlen et al. 1988).

The early recognition and surgical removal of dysplastic nevi has become a major concern of dermatologists and clinical oncologists in melanoma prevention. It is certainly not my intention, therefore, to belittle the outstanding merits of Dr. Lynch and Dr. Clark when I question one aspect of their work, namely the assumption of a single gene causing the association of dysplastic nevi and malignant melanoma.

Are Dysplastic Nevi a Dichotomic or Continuous Trait?

The original hypothesis underlying the so-called dysplastic nevus syndrome was that dysplastic nevi are uncommon and seen only in association with familial melanomas. As already pointed out, it is now well established that dysplastic nevi are, however, very frequent lesions.

Sporadic dysplastic nevi outnumber familial dysplastic nevi by a factor of at least 10:1. This should confirm that dysplastic nevi do not form a rare, monogenic syndrome. However, instead of doubting the existence of a distinct dysplastic nevus syndrome as a single gene entity, its proponents described a second syndrome, namely the *sporadic dysplastic nevus syndrome* (Elder et al. 1980).

In the mean time, it has even been suggested that there are five different types of dysplastic nevus syndromes (Kraemer et al. 1983). In reality, the five proposed syndromes are not distinct clinical entities but different risk categories of the same entity, and the major criterion for classification is the number of family members having dysplastic nevi and/or melanomas.

Though a classification into different categories having different risks for malignant melanoma may be very helpful for the clinician and for the epidemiologist, it is artificial from the viewpoint of mendelian genetics. In a single-gene disorder the risk of developing a certain phenotype is constant. Risks that are dependent on the number of family members already affected therefore strongly indicate polygenic inheritance (Happle et al. 1982; Traupe and Macher 1988).

The debate on the inheritance of malignant melanoma and its precursor lesions centers on the claim that at least two and perhaps even five different syndromes can be distinguished, i.e., that dysplastic nevi are a dichotomic phenotype. Is it justified to separate a disease into two or even five different entities, just because it appears in a pattern in some families, while it is sporadic in most cases? This kind of subclassification is done only in tumor genetics, not in other genetic subdisciplines. For example, nobody seriously suggests that

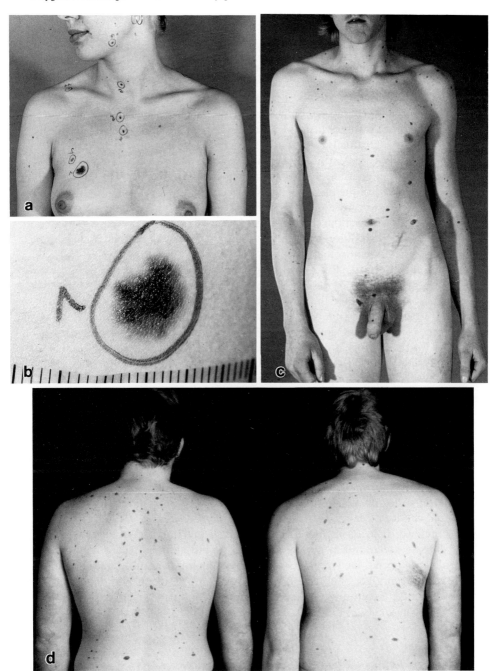

Fig. 1a-d. Dysplastic nevi. **a** multiple sporadic dysplastic nevi; **b** close-up of one nevus showing irregular and ill-defined borders and a dark-brown varied pigmentation on a pink background (same patient as in **a**; **c** multiple dysplastic nevi also involving areas not exposed to the sun in a patient with a negative family history; **d** familial occurrence of dysplastic nevi in two brothers with negative family history for melanoma. (**a** and **b** from Traupe et al. 1989)

psoriasis is a different disease when occurring sporadically in one patient than when presenting in a family.

The readiness of at least some geneticists to accept a dichotomic view of dysplastic nevi and malignant melanoma may in part be due to the fact that some uncommon monogenic tumor syndromes do exist. Most of the proven monogenic tumor syndromes have, however, additional features distinguishing them from the normal solitary and sporadic type. Thus, the basal cell carcinoma nevus syndrome is not just the clustering of multiple basal cell carcinomas in a family, but has further distinctive and pathognomonic features such as facial dysmorphia, jaw cysts, calcification of the falx cerebri, and pits on palms and soles. In recent years familial retinoblastoma has become the outstanding model of tumor genetics because of the loss of an antioncogene on the long arm of chromosome 13 at q14 (reviewed by Sager 1986). However, even the familial type of retinoblastoma differs from the sporadic type by showing far more frequent bilateral involvement. Such differences are not found between the familial and sporadic dysplastic nevus syndrome.

On the contrary, clinical, histologic, and epidemiologic evidence indicates that dysplastic nevi represent a continuous or quantitative trait. Most histopathologists will agree that there are continuous transitions between ordinary and dysplastic nevi and between dysplastic nevi and malignant melanomas (Happle et al. 1982). Moreover, there is not a single clinical or histologic feature that is in itself specific or predictive of dysplastic nevi. Steijlen et al. (1988) established that at least two major and one minor criteria have to be combined to reach a reasonable efficacy for histologic diagnosis.

Another crucial point supporting the notion of dysplastic nevi as a quantitative or continuous trait is the fact that the total number of nevus cell nevi is an important risk factor for both dysplastic nevi and malignant melanoma (reviewed by Welkovich et al. 1989). Holly et al. (1987) were able to show that the relative risk for melanoma rises from 1.6 with 11–25 nevus cell nevi to 9.8 with 100 or more nevus cell nevi. Such a correlation is not confined to sporadic melanoma, but is also present in the melanoma families. Kraemer and Greene (1985) found that in the NIH series of melanoma families, people with more than 100 nevi had a 19-fold chance of developing melanoma than *affected* relatives with fewer nevi. In other words, even in these highly selected melanoma families, the risk of developing melanoma is not constant for the individual affected members, as would be expected for a monogenic trait, but depends to a considerable extent on the variable number of precursor lesions present. This inconstant risk is a strong indication for a continuous or quantitative trait and can be best explained by a polygenic model (Happle 1989; Traupe and Happle 1990).

Excessive Mutation Rates Indicate a Polygenic Model

It is a well-accepted law of population genetics that there is a genetic equilibrium between newly arising and eliminated mutations (for review, see Stern 1974).

Otherwise, some diseases would become exceedingly frequent or would disappear completely. In general, the ratio of eliminated to newly arising mutations is 1:1. The number of eliminated mutations can be calculated indirectly according to the Haldane formula. For a dominant disease the Haldane formula is $\mu = 0.5 \times (1-F) \times i$. In this equation μ is the mutation rate, F the reproductive fitness and i is the incidence of the trait. The reproductive fitness, i.e., the fitness of reproduction compared with the general population, is surprisingly high (as shown by Bale and Tucker 1990) — probably close to 99%. The incidence of the trait is about 0.06% since 10% of all melanomas are familial and the overall incidence of melanoma is about 0.6%. If we accept that these figures reflect the real situation only very few mutations are eliminated and the calculation gives a figure for the mutation rate of $\mu = 3 \times 10^{-6}$.

We can now estimate the mutation rate derived directly from the phenotype actually observed. In dominant diseases, sporadic occurrence is interpreted as a new mutation. Since several population surveys indicate an incidence of the trait in the range 2%–10%, this would translate into absurdly high mutation rates of between 1×10^{-2} and 5×10^{-2}. It has been argued that the directly observed mutation rate should not be derived from the incidence of sporadic dysplastic nevi, but from the lower incidence of dysplastic nevi in association with malignant melanoma (Bale and Tucker 1990). We do not share this view because it again suggests a separation between "true" dysplastic nevi and those which are highly unlikely to become malignant (Traupe and Happle 1990). However, even then the mutation rate remains abnormally high. It is generally agreed that about 30%–50% of all sporadic melanoma patients display dysplastic nevi and the corresponding mutation rate would then be in the range of $\mu = 9 \times 10^{-4}$ to 1.5×10^{-3} (Table 2).

It can be concluded that mutation rate estimates derived directly are much higher (in the range of 9×10^{-4} to 5×10^{-2}) than the mutation rates calculated indirectly according to Haldane's formula ($\mu = 3 \times 10^{-6}$). In other words, newly arising mutations are at least 100 times more frequent than eliminated mutations. This apparent lack of a genetic equilibrium is not compatible with autosomal dominant inheritance and strongly indicates a polygenic model (Traupe et al. 1989).

Single Factors Involved in the Polygenic Predisposition to Malignant Melanoma and Dysplastic Nevi

A number of genes and chromosomes are probably involved in the polygenic predisposition to malignant melanoma and dysplastic nevi:

(1) Major gene(s) controlling nevus cell counts
(2) Ethnogene(s) responsible for pigmentary characteristics such as skin complexion and hair color
(3) Tumor repressor gene (antioncogene) possibly located on chromosome 6q

Table 2. Calculation and comparison of mutation rates of the dysplastic nevus syndrome

Calculation of eliminated mutations with Haldane's formula

μ = $0.5 (1 - F) i$, where
μ = mutation rate
F = reproductive fitness = 99%
   (data according to Bale and Tucker 1990)
i = incidence of the trait = 6×10^{-4}
   since 1 out of 10 melanomas is familial
μ = $0.5 (1 - 0.99) 6 \times 10^{-4} = 3 \times 10^{-6}$

Directly derived mutation rate of newly arising mutations

a) Based on incidence of sporadic dysplastic nevi in the range 2%–10%
   μ = $0.5 \times i_a$
   μ = $0.5 \times 2 \times 10^{-2}$ to $10 \times 10^{-2} = 1 \times 10^{-2}$ to 5×10^{-2}
b) Based on incidence of sporadic dysplastic nevi associated with sporadic melanoma
   1. incidence of sporadic melanoma = 6×10^{-3}
   2. incidence of sporadic DN associated with melanoma (30%–50%):
      i_b = 0.3 to $0.5 \times 6 \times 10^{-3} = 1.8$ to 3.0×10^{-3}
      μ = 0.5×1.8 to $3.0 \times 10^{-3} = 9 \times 10^{-4}$ to 1.5×10^{-3}

Comparison of mutation rates

Directly observed: $\mu = 9 \times 10^{-4}$ to 5×10^{-2}
Indirectly calculated: $\mu = 3 \times 10^{-6}$

Conclusion: Lack of a genetic equilibrium between newly arising and eliminated mutations (ratio 100:1 instead of 1:1)

(4) *Possible*: Gene for complementation group D mutation of xeroderma pigmentosum
(5) *Possible*: Linkage with chromosome 1p markers (in one of four studies)

The relationship between the number of ordinary nevus cell nevi and the risk for malignant melanoma has already been discussed. On the basis of twin studies, Siemens (1924) concluded that despite environmental influences nevus cell counts are under genetic control. The existence of a major gene controlling nevus cell counts can also be inferred from a unique clinical case observation. Sterry and Christophers (1988) reported a 59-year-old man who displayed numerous pigmented skin lesions including a large number of ordinary nevus cell nevi, several dysplastic nevi, and two malignant melanomas in a quadrant distribution. The mosaic manifestation of pigmented lesions in this patient can be best explained by a somatic mutation during early embryogenesis affecting a gene responsible for mole counts. Thus, there is a strong case for a major gene or (less likely) a set of genes controlling nevus counts in the predisposition to melanoma.

A second gene or a set of genes involved in malignant melanoma and its precursor lesions concern those determining hair color and skin complexion. Epidemiologic studies underline the importance of pigmentary characteristics (Holman and Armstrong 1984; Holly et al. 1987). It has been shown that these pigmentary characteristics reflect ethnic differences (Rampen 1988). It is well known that hair color is a polygenic trait and determined by at least three different genes.

A third major gene (or possibly even a set of genes) is a tumor-repressor gene (antioncogene). The existence of an antioncogene is indicated by marked racial differences in melanoma incidence (reviewed by Crombie 1979). The lowest melanoma incidence is found among American Indians. The incidence among people of Spanish descent is higher, but still much lower than among people with an Anglo-Saxon/Celtic ethnic background. Interestingly, the melanoma rate is relatively high in South-American populations which are largely a mixture of Spanish or Portuguese and American Indians. In these mixed populations melanoma incidence is in the range of that found in Caucasians with an Anglo-Saxon/Celtic background (Crombie 1979). This "experiment of Nature" reminds us of a similar situation in the platyfish/swordtail melanoma system where crossing experiments eliminate tumor repressor genes (see following section).

Cytogenetic clues support the presence of an antioncogene for melanoma which may be located on the long arm of chromosome 6 (Pathak et al. 1983; Herlyn et al. 1985) the distal segment of which is often translocated to various other chromosomes. Very recently, Trent et al. (1990) demonstrated that introduction of a normal chromosome 6 into melanoma cell lines reverts the tumorigenicity of these cells in mice.

There is one example where melanoma is consistently caused by a single gene, namely a certain type of *xeroderma pigmentosum*: the complementation group D mutation (Jung et al. 1986). This subtype is a very uncommon autosomal recessive disorder having an incidence of about 1×10^{-6}. A look at the Hardy-Weinberg law shows that the incidence of heterozygous gene carriers for this disorder is 2×10^{-3} or in other words one in 500 of the general population. It is conceivable, but not proven, that this gene, which has not been mapped so far, contributes to the incidence of malignant melanoma also in heterozygous gene carriers.

Linkage studies performed in melanoma families have so far been disappointing or have given very contradictory results. The NIH group recently claimed linkage between distal chromosome 1p markers and the gene for the dysplastic nevus syndrome (Bale et al. 1989). In contrast, in a very large patient group studied in the Netherlands by the Leiden group the "Dutch" gene for the dysplastic nevus syndrome could be definitely excluded from this region of chromosome 1 (van Haeringen et al. 1989). At the recent workshop on genetic epidemiology of cancer held at the German Cancer Research Center in Heidelberg, 22 and 23 January 1990, Dr. Lynch, of Omaha, Neb. USA, and Dr. Lisa Cannon-Albright, of Salt Lake City, Utah, USA, briefly mentioned that they were also unable to find linkage with 1p markers in their families. In my opinion the apparent inability to find a reliable linkage despite painstaking efforts reflects the presence of more than one major gene in the families tested. Successful linkage analysis may therefore require a new approach (see Conclusion).

Melanoma in the Platyfish/Swordtail System:
An Animal Model for Polygenic Control of Melanoma

When mentioning the increased incidence of melanoma in human racial hybrid populations in South America reference to an analogous situation in the platyfish/swordtail system was made. This system is one of the best-studied animal models of tumorigenesis. It has been established beyond doubt that melanoma formation is under the control of at least four genes in this system (Anders and Anders 1978; Schwab 1987). An X-linked tumor gene and at least three autosomal tumor repressor genes have been identified (Ahuja et al. 1980; Schwab 1987). The platyfish *Xiphophorus* has spotted pigmentation of the dorsal fin and contains both the tumor gene and several repressor genes. The swordtail *Xiphophorus helleri* has no pigmented spots and contains neither tumor nor repressor genes. When the two fish are crossed a hybrid develops which shows an enhancement of pigmentation. If this hybrid is backcrossed with a nonpigmented *Xiphophorus helleri*, 50% of the offspring show a normal helleri phenotype with no tumor genes, but possibly repressor genes, and the remaining 50% show melanoma which can have a broad range and corresponding to what we call a "continuous" trait (Fig. 2). In this beautiful animal model of polygenic control of melanoma formation it was recently possible to clone the X-linked tumor gene

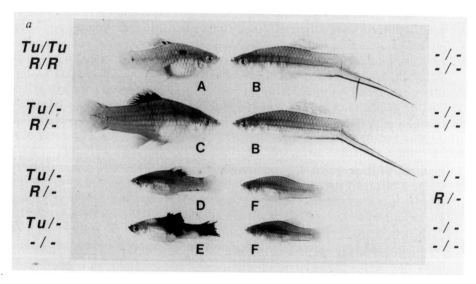

Fig. 2. Polygenic control of melanoma in the platyfish (*Xiphophorus maculatus*)/swordtail (*Xiphophorus helleri*) system. *X. maculatus A* containing both tumor and repressor genes is crossed with *X. helleri B* lacking these genes. The resulting offspring *C* shows enhancement of the reported dorsal phenotype. *C* is backcrossed with *X. helleri B*. 50% of the offspring of this mating develop melanoma (*D* and *E*) due to elimination of tumor repressor genes, while 50% are phenotypically like the parental *X. helleri* strain *F*. Courtesy of Dr. Wittbrodt, from Wittbrodt et al. (1989)

which shows considerable sequence homology with the epidermal growth-factor receptor and represents a further receptor tyrosine kinase (Wittbrodt et al. 1989).

Conclusions

In this review the prevailing dogma that the dysplastic nevus syndrome is a single gene disorder is questioned, and a polygenic concept is proposed instead. Three major genetic components involved in the control of dysplastic nevi and malignant melanoma have been elaborated:

(1) A gene or set of genes responsible for pigmentary characteristics,
(2) a gene or set of genes controlling the number of ordinary nevus cell nevi, and
(3) a gene or set of antioncogenes (tumor repressor genes).

In addition to these three major components, further minor genes may exert a modifying influence. A successful strategy to identify one of the three postulated major genes with use of DNA markers and linkage analysis could be to test within ethnically homogeneous populations, thus eliminating the racial factor. Moreover, I suggest dismantling the dysplastic nevus syndrome phenotype, i.e., looking at melanoma, dysplastic nevi, and nevus cell counts separately. Finally, even in melanoma families the presence of dysplastic nevi in a given family member by no means proves the presence of the major melanoma gene and it may be wise to confine linkage analysis to family members affected with melanoma and obligate carriers of the presumed melanoma susceptibility gene.

Acknowledgments. Dr. Rudolf Happle and Dr. Hans-Hilger Ropers, both of Nijmegen, and Dr. Lisa A. Cannon-Albright of Salt Lake City are thanked for discussion of the topic.

References

Ahuja MR, Schwab M, Anders F (1980) Linkage between a regulatory locus for melanoma cell differentiation and esterase locus in *Xiphophorus*. J Hered 7:403–407

Anders A, Anders F (1978) Etiology of cancer as studied in the platyfish-swordtail system. Biochem Biophys Acta 516:61–95

Anderson DE (1971) Clinical characteristics of the genetic variety of cutaneous melanoma in man. Cancer 28:721–725

Bale SJ, Chakravarti A, Greene MH (1986) Cutaneous malignant melanoma and familial dysplastic nevi: evidence for autosomal dominance and pleiotropy. Am J Hum Genet 38:188–196

Bale SJ, Dracopoli NC, Tucker MA, Clark WH Jr, Fraser MC, Stanger BZ, Green P, Donis-Keller H, Housman DE, Greene MH (1989) Mapping the gene for hereditary cutaneous malignant melanoma-dysplastic nevus to chromosome 1p. N Engl J Med 320:1367–1372

Bale SJ, Tucker MA (1990) Mutation rate estimates in hereditary cutaneous malignant melanoma/dysplastic nevi (letter). Am J Med Genet 35:293–294

Bergman W, Palan A, Went LN (1986) Clinical and genetic studies in six Dutch kindreds with the dysplastic nevus syndrome. Ann Hum Genet 50:249–258

Cawley EP (1952) Genetic aspects of malignant melanoma. Arch Dermatol 65:440–450

Clark WH Jr, Reimer DR, Greene M, Ainsworth AM, Mastrangelo MJ (1978) Origin of familial malignant melanomas from heritable melanocytic lesions. "The B-K mole syndrome". Arch Dermatol 114:732–738

Crombie IK (1979) Racial differences in melanoma incidence. Br J Cancer 40:185–193

Elder DE, Goldman LI, Goldman SC, Greene MH, Clark WH Jr (1980) Dysplastic nevus syndrome. A phenotypic association of sporadic cutaneous malignant melanoma. Cancer 46:1787–1794

Happle R (1989) Gregor Mendel und die dysplastischen Nävi. Hautarzt 40:70–76

Happle R, Traupe H (1982) Polygene Vererbung der familiären malignen Melanome. Hautarzt 33:106–111

Happle R, Traupe H, Vakilzadeh F, Macher E (1982) Arguments in favor of a polygenic inheritance of precursor nevi. J Am Acad Dermatol 6:540–543

Herlyn M, Thurin J, Balaban G, Bennicelli JL, Herlyn DE, Bondi E, Guerry DP, Nowell P, Clark W, Koprowski H (1985) Characteristics of cultured human melanocytes isolated from different stages of tumor progression. Cancer Res 451:5670–5676

Holly EA, Kelly JW, Shpall SN, Chiu SH (1987) Number of melanocytic nevi as a major risk factor for malignant melanoma. J Am Acad Dermatol 17:459–468

Holman CDJ, Armstrong BK (1984) Pigmentary traits, ethnic origin, benign nevi, and family history as risk factors for cutaneous malignant melanoma. J Natl Cancer Inst 72:257–266

Jung EG, Bohnert E, Fischer E (1986) Heterogeneity of xeroderma pigmentosum (XP); variability and stability within and between the complementation groups C, D, E, I and variants. Photodermatol 3:125–132

Kraemer KH, Greene MH (1985) Dysplastic nevus syndrome. Familial and sporadic precursors of cutaneous melanoma. Dermatol Clin 3:225–237

Kraemer KH, Greene MH, Tarone R, Elder DE, Clark WH, Guerry D (1983) Dysplastic nevi and cutaneous melanoma risk. Lancet II:1076–1077

Lynch HT, Frichot BC, Lynch JF (1978) Familial atypical multiple mole melanoma syndrome. J Med Genet 15:352–356

Miller TR, Pack GT (1962) The familial aspect of malignant melanoma. Arch Dermatol 86:35–39

National Institutes of Health (NIH) (1984) Precursor to malignant melanoma. National Institutes of Health Concensus Development Conference statement, Oct 24–26, 1983. J Am Acad Dermatol 10:683–688

Pathak S, Drwinga HL, Hsu TC (1983) Involvement of chromosome 6 in rearrangements in human malignant melanoma cell lines. Cytogenet Cell Genet 36:573–579

Rampen FHJ (1988) Nevocytic nevi and skin complexion. Dermatologica 176:111–114

Sager R (1986) Genetic suppression of tumor formation. A new frontier in cancer research. Cancer Res 46:1573–1580

Salamon T, Schnyder UW, Storck H (1963) A contribution to the question of heredity of malignant melanomas. Dermatologica 126:65–75

Schwab M (1987) Oncogenes and tumor suppressor genes in Xiphophorus. Trends Genet 3:38–42

Sherrington R, Brynjolfsson J, Petursson H, Potter M, Dudleston K, Barraclough B, Wasmuth J, Dobbs M, Gurling H (1988) Localization of a susceptibility locus for schizophrenia on chromosome 5. Nature 336:164–167

Siemens HW (1924) Die Zwillingspathologie. Ihre Bedeutung, ihre Methodik, ihre bisherigen Ergebnisse. Springer, Berlin Heidelberg New York, pp 24–25, 47–48

Solomon E, Voss R, Hall V, Bodmer WF, Jass JR, Jeffreys AJ, Lucibello FC, Patel I, Rider SH (1987) Chromosome 5 allele loss in human colorectal carcinomas. Nature 328:616–619

Steijlen PM, Bergman W, Hermans J, Scheffer E, Van Vloten WA, Ruiter DJ (1988) The efficacy of histopathological criteria required for diagnosing dysplastic nevi. Histopathology 12:289–300

Stern C (1974) Principles of human genetics, 3rd edn. Freeman, San Francisco, pp 552–580

Sterry W, Christophers E (1988) Quadrant distribution of dysplastic nevus syndrome. Arch Dermatol 124:926–929

Traupe H, Happle R (1990) The dysplastic nevus "syndrome" is not a dichotomic, but a continuous phenotype. Am J Med Genet 35:295–296

Traupe H, Macher E (1988) Classical and molecular genetics of malignant melanoma and dysplastic nevi. In: Elwood JM (ed) Melanoma and nevi. Incidence, interrelationships and implications. Pigment Cell, vol 9. Karger, Basel, pp 77–94

Traupe H, Macher E, Hamm H, Happle R (1989) Mutation rate estimates are not compatible with autosomal dominant inheritance of the dysplastic nevus "syndrome". Am J Med Genet 32:155–157

Tucker MA (1988) Individuals at high risk of melanoma. In: Elwood JM (ed) Melanoma and nevi. Incidence, interrelationships and implications. Pigment Cell, vol 9. Karger, Basel, pp 95–109

Trent ZM, Stanbridge EZ, Mc Bride HL et al. (1990) Tumorigenicity in human melanoma cell lines controlled by introduction of human chromosome 6. Science 247:568–571

Van Haeringen A, Bergman W, Nelen MR, Van der Kooij-Meijs E, Hendrikse I, Wijnen JT, Meera Khan PM, Klasen EC, Frants RR (1989) Exclusion of the dysplastic nevus syndrome (DNS) locus from the short arm of chromosome 1 by linkage studies in Dutch families. Genomics 5:61–64

Wallace DC, Exton LA, McLeod GRC (1971) Genetic factor in malignant melanoma. Cancer 27:1262–1266

Welkovich B, Landthaler M, Schmoeckel C, Braun-Falco O (1989) Anzahl und Verteilung von Nävuszellnävi bei Patienten mit malignem Melanom. Hautarzt 40:630–635

Wittbrodt J, Adam D, Malitschek B, Mäueler W, Raulf F, Telling A, Robertson SM, Schartl M (1989) Novel putative receptor tyrosine kinase encoded by the melanoma-inducing Tu locus in Xiphophorus. Nature 341:415–421

Genetic Epidemiology and the Familial Atypical Multiple Mole Melanoma Syndrome*

H.T. Lynch[1] and R.M. Fusaro[2]

Introduction

Cutaneous malignant melanoma (CMM) has been increasing in many of the western industrialized nations at a frequency which exceeds that of any other form of cancer (Magnus 1987). This disease has reached epidemic proportions among patients with light pigmentation residing in the southwestern United States and in several southern nations of the world (Crombie 1979; Green and Siskind 1983). For example, in Australia, the annual incidence of CMM is 32.7 per 100 000 individuals (Green and Siskind 1983).

Host factors, as these apply to pigmentation as well as to the presence of CMM in one or more of the patients' close relatives, are extremely important in the comprehension of its etiology (Lynch and Fusaro 1982). It is noteworthy that there is a 12-fold increased risk for CMM among patients with one or more first degree relatives with CMM when compared with patients who are members of families lacking CMM (Duggleby et al. 1981). Among individuals with an initial CMM, the risk for secondary primary CMM is increased 900-fold (Kopf et al. 1986). More systematic research investigating a likely relationship between a genetic predisposition to malignant melanoma and environmental interaction is needed. This phenomenon has been advanced in terms of a unifying etiologic hypothesis by Lynch and Fusaro (1986; Fig. 1).

Historical Development of the FAMMM Syndrome

Norris (1820) is credited with what may possibly be the first description of a family with the hereditary form of CMM which was consonant with the familial atypical multiple mole melanoma (FAMMM) syndrome. In this family, melanoma appeared in a 59-year-old male. Thirty years prior to his death, his father had died

* This study is supported by NIH grant # 1 RO1 CA47429 and a grant from the Nebraska Cancer and Smoking Disease Research Program
[1] Department of Preventive Medicine/Public Health, Creighton University School of Medicine, Omaha, NE 68178, USA
[2] Departments of Medicine-Dermatology, University of Nebraska Medical Center, Omaha, NE 68105, USA and Creighton University School of Medicine, Omaha, NE 68178, USA

H.T. Lynch and P. Tautu (Eds.)
Recent Progress
in the Genetic Epidemiology of Cancer
© Springer-Verlag Berlin Heidelberg 1991

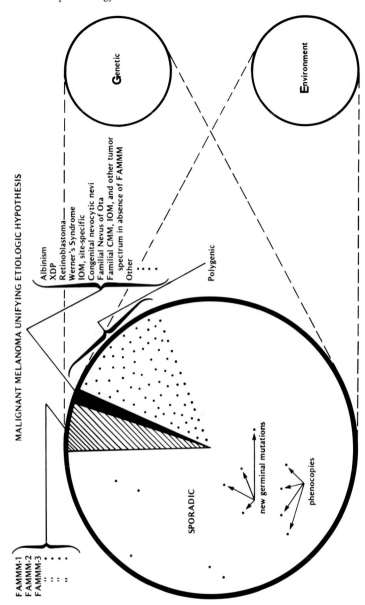

Fig. 1. The unifying etiologic hypothesis for the extant heterogeneity in hereditary malignant melanoma. *FAMMM*, familial atypical multiple mole melanoma syndrome (suffixes indicate heterogeneous forms); *XDP*, xeroderma pigmentosum; *IOM*, intraocular malignant melanoma, site specific; *CMM*, cutaneous malignant melanoma. (From Lynch and Fusaro 1986)

of a similar disease. Reportedly, a surgeon who had attended this patient's father observed that he had many moles on various parts of his body and that his children, including the index patient, also had multiple moles. The surgeon suggested that the disease was hereditary.

There were no further reports of familial malignant melanoma until the contemporary study by Cawley (1952) who described CMMs in a father and two of his three children. Lynch et al. (1978) and Clark et al. (1978) described the FAMMM syndrome simultaneously in 1978. This disorder has also been named the hereditary dysplastic nevus syndrome (HDNS). These terms will be used interchangeably in this paper.

The FAMMM syndrome (HDNS) is characterized by an autosomal dominantly inherited predisposition to multiple atypical nevi (AN) and CMMs. However, as in virtually *all* hereditary disorders, particularly those showing an autosomal dominant inheritance pattern, there is variable expressivity of the phenotype, reduced penetrance of the gene, and problems in the interpretation of phenocopies and genocopies. Therefore, any classic, clinical genetic definition, as we have provided, must be tempered by these potentially limiting genetic obfuscations.

In the paper by Clark et al. (1978), the disorder was initially referred to as the B-K mole syndrome. A litany of names for this disorder(s) have appeared in the literature: e.g., HDNS (Elder et al. 1980) and the large atypical nevus syndrome (LANS) (Bondi et al. 1981), to name just two. However, Lynch and Fusaro have considered FAMMM to be appropriately descriptive of the syndrome and have steadfastly adhered to this terminology. Interestingly, investigators have now come almost full circle in the matter of nomenclature, as evidenced by the latest suggested terminology, namely, "atypical mole syndrome," as designated by Kopf et al. (1990). This latter designation places the diagnosis of the FAMMM syndrome on the pivotal criterion of the histologic confirmation of the clinical presence of the cutaneous atypical nevus phenotype. This reliance on only one (histologic confirmation of AN) of the three cutaneous phenotypic expressions (presence of AN, the total mole count of the patient, and the presence of malignant melanoma) of the FAMMM syndrome is fraught with a high rate of error. As will be discussed later, AN occur in normal individuals.

Genetic Epidemiology of CMM

Surprisingly, there has been limited investigation of the etiologic role of environmental interaction in the FAMMM syndrome. For example, in spite of the prodigious evidence for the significance of solar radiation exposure in the etiology of CMM, we are not aware of any clinical evidence showing the effect of sunlight exposure on AN or CMM in the FAMMM syndrome.

A study of keen interest in the genetic epidemiology of CMM is that of Roser et al. (1989) on the manner in which genetically enhanced susceptibility to ultraviolet (UV) radiation may play a crucial etiologic role in the evolution of

CMM at the laboratory level. These researchers studied skin fibroblasts from 26 patients with CMM and controls. They used the micronucleus (MN) test and sister chromatid exchange (SCE) following UV radiation. SCE and MN formation were then employed as investigational parameters for the detection of UV-induced genotoxic damage in the individual cell strains. Results disclosed "...that the UV-induced level of MN was significantly increased in CMM patients ($p = 0.0005$), being most pronounced in the familial cases ($p = 0.0001$). Ultraviolet-induced SCE was also elevated in CMM patients ($p = 0.001$), but there was no difference between familial and nonfamilial cases. The present findings indicate that genetic predisposition contributes to the development of CMM in a subset of CMM patients and may be due to an enhanced susceptibility to UV light." This methodologic approach needs to be pursued in well-defined FAMMM kindreds.

Prototype Clinical/Genetic Model of the FAMMM Syndrome

Our original FAMMM kindred (Fig. 2) has been followed by us for almost a quarter century [Lynch and Krush 1968; Lynch et al. 1978, 1980, 1981, 1983, 1985). This single kindred has provided us with the unique opportunity to extensively study the genetics, pathology, and natural history of the FAMMM syndrome. Clearly, the cutaneous phenotypes in the proband (Fig. 3) and the evolution of AN in his daughter (Fig. 4) depicts these findings in high relief. However, during the past decade, we have learned that variation in all facets of the phenotypes must be meticulously scrutinized so that the best posits of the clinical and pathologic study can be used for securing confidence in diagnosis.

Clinical Findings

The cutaneous manifestations of the FAMMM syndrome are such that there is a spectrum of clinical findings which range from the florid expression of many large AN, with the individual having moles too numerous to count and with or without CMM, through the affected individual with one or two AN and a normal mole count (i.e., the patient has approximately the normal number of 20–30 total nevi), to the other end of the clinical spectrum in which the kindred member has no nevi but has CMM. The classic expression of the cutaneous findings are summarized in Table 1.

The clinical recognition of the classic FAMMM adult patient for the well-trained clinician is a reflex visual response that takes no more than a fleeting glance (Fig. 3). The recognition of the minimal expression of the AN is a most difficult problem and may be impossible clinically because of the spectrum of the expression of the FAMMM phenotypes due to the variable expressivity, the incomplete gene penetrance, and the heterogeneity of this hereditary precan-

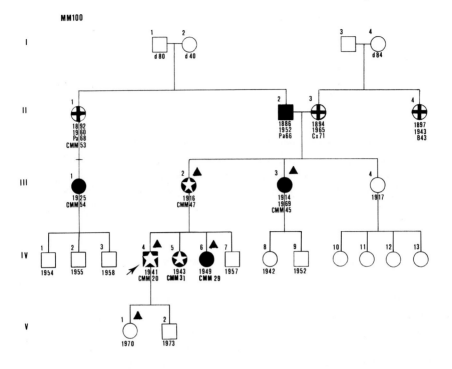

Legend

⟋ Proband

□ or ○ Male or female unaffected by cancer

1 ₂ Pedigree code

■ ● Cancer verified by pathology

1924 1957 Year of birth

1970 1963 Year of death

CMM20 Pa66 Cancer site and age, initial diagnosis

⊞ ● Cancer verified by death certificate or medical record

◘ ◉ Multiple primary cancer

▲ Pathologically confirmed abnormal compound nevi

■ Breast

PA Pancreas

CX Cervix

CMM Cutaneous malignant melanoma

Fig. 2. This pedigree shows the proband with multiple primary CMMs (13 in over a 25-year period) and occurrence of pancreatic carcinoma in putative obligate gene carriers. Since the submission of this manuscript two members of this pedigree have developed a malignancy. Individual III-2 has developed an adenocarcinoma of the pancreas at age 73 and subsequently died within the year. This represents the third member of this family to die of an adenocarcinoma of the pancreas. All three of these members had the cutaneous phenotype (III-2) or were obligate gene carriers (II-1 and II-2). Individual IV-4, who as a child had dysplastic nevi and an increased number of nevi on her body, has developed a malignant melanoma at age 20

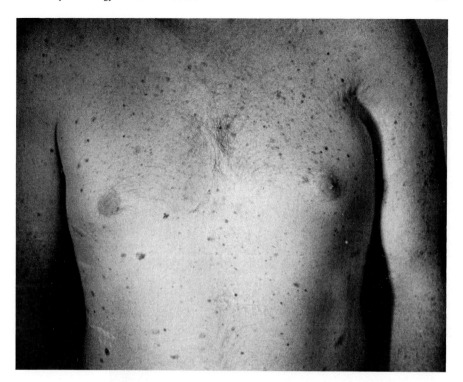

Fig. 3. Front view of the proband (IV-4) from Fig. 2. Note the presence of multiple moles, several of which are strikingly atypical (From Lynch et al. 1980)

cerous syndrome. In addition, the minimal expression of atypical nevi blends into the clinical appearance of the banal or common nevus. In older members of a pedigree, the recognition of the clinical phenotype of AN is difficult since all nevi tend to regress with age, but in the FAMMM syndrome the nevi appear to regress at a slower rate and persist through the fourth and fifth decades of life before further regression takes place in the seventh and eight decades (unpublished observations). We do not regularly see the clinical phenotypes of many nevi, and large numbers of atypical nevi of the FAMMM syndrome in the seventh or later decades of life of our patients with this syndrome.

Many prepubertal children from FAMMM kindreds will have total mole counts greater than those seen in normal children (unpublished observations). Atypical nevi are present at an early age in some patients but again they have not been systematically documented because of the reticence of doing routine excision of AN in children and the rarity of malignant melanoma in children of FAMMM kindreds. When AN appear in children, they are indistinguishable clinically from normal nevi. It is only when they reach 4–6 mm in diameter that they begin to acquire the classic phenotypic characteristics that allow them to be recognized. What is recognizable in these children is that they develop nevi at an

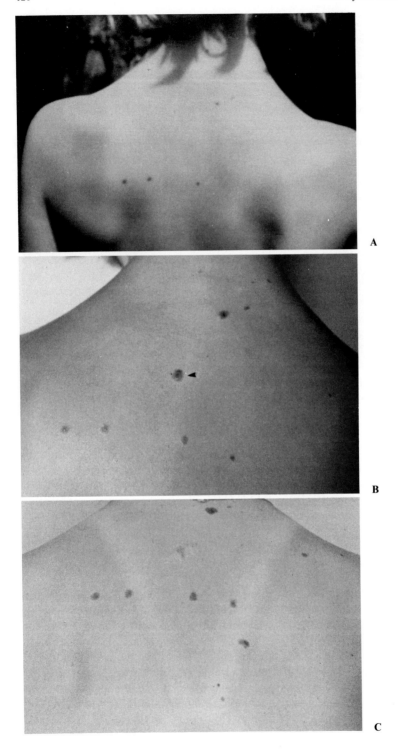

A

B

C

Table 1. Clinical characteristics of the cutaneous FAMMM phenotypes

Characteristics	Clinical expression
Number of total nevi (both AN and normal nevi)	Greater than normal count: often 50–100 or more, with lesions of all sizes and shapes (heterogeneous) Unknown: percentage of normal vs AN The lower limits of number have not been defined
Size of AN	From 5 mm or greater The lower limits of size recognition unknown
Border of AN	Serpiginous or irregular with color leakage (fading) into surrounding skin. Border may be sharp and oval or round with no pigment fading at periphery
Color of AN	Variegate: red, tan, brown, and even almost black; individual lesions may be only one color
Contour of AN	Usually macular but often raised centrally with the surface occasionally mammillated (fine cobblestones)
Anatomic location of AN	Trunk and proximal extremities, but scalp in both sexes and legs in females
Age of recognition of AN	Puberty; description of AN in children is limited but recognizable AN (>4 mm) have been reported
Rate of change and time span	Nevi usually start appearing early in the first decade of life, with number greater than normal. New nevi continue to appear into the 4th and 5th decades of life. Both normal-appearing nevi and especially AN increase in size and change color. These nevi regress in the 7th and 8th decades of life
Normal nevi in FAMMM	Present, but in greater number than normal; however, the extent and definition has not been determined
Malignant melanoma	Presence of CMM with other phenotypes of AN and/or increased total mole count, but CMM can be present in the absence of any nevi. CMMs appear after puberty

early age and in greater numbers than in normal children and, in addition, may develop AN at an early age (Fig. 4; Lynch et al. 1985).

The recognition of the FAMMM patient in the context of the kindred setting is established when the first and second degree relatives of the kindred show the classic clinical phenotypic findings of the FAMMM syndrome with an autosomal dominant pattern of inheritance. The clinical diagnosis in relatives can be difficult when each of the characteristics listed in Table 1 is minimally expressed. The

◀ **Fig. 4. A** The proband's daughter at age 5 years. Note three nevi in a row. **B** The patient at age 8 years. The three nevi are now four in a row. The large atypical nevus (*arrow*) developed since last photo and was removed for histologic examination. **C** The patient at age 13 years. The four nevi are larger and dark in pigmentation. Other nevi have also increased in size and pigmentation (From Lynch et al. 1985)

important clinical phenotype to be measured in the patient is the total number of all nevi. Another important phenotypic characteristic is the presence of AN and their total number. The third clinical phenotype of note is the presence of malignant melanoma. The latter may be present in the absence of any nevi. When evaluating a kindred member, all of the cutaneous phenotypic characteristics must be documented before a final presumptive diagnostic decision can be considered. Even then, each kindred member must be considered with respect to his immediate first and second degree relatives, as the individual can be an obligate gene carrier with no cutaneous phenotypic expression of the FAMMM syndrome.

Histologic Findings of AN

Until recently, it was assumed that the clinical presence of AN was presumptively diagnostic for FAMMM patients as these nevi were only present in patients with the syndrome or in the sporadic variant. In studies of large FAMMM kindreds in Utah, Piepkorn et al. (1989) have shown that 53% of spouse controls in FAMMM pedigrees had clinically a few AN (confirmed histologically). The clinical diagnosis of AN is considered to be confirmed by the microscopic presence of the following histologic characteristics:

(a) architectural atypia,
(b) cellular atypia,
(c) stromal fibroplasia with angiogenesis, and
(d) a chronic lymphocytic infiltrate.

These histologic findings are identical in patients with either the FAMMM syndrome or the sporadic AN variant. Steijlen et al. (1988) used various histologic features seen in dysplastic nevi, and found by discriminant analysis that the most discriminating histologic elements for the diagnosis of AN were, in decreasing order, the presence of dust-like melanin pigment, irregular nests of melanocytes, markedly increased junctional activity, and melanocytic nuclei larger than or as large as overlying keratinocytes. The efficacy of any single diagnostic feature of the many histologic characteristics of dysplastic nevi was limited due to low sensitivity, low specificity, or low predictive value, but when combinations of two or more of the four criteria cited above were used, a high degree of discrimination could be reached that would separate AN in FAMMM patients from AN in a normal group of controls.

The minimal expression of each of these characteristic histologic findings blends into the classic activated junctional nevi of normal individuals. Thus, the histologic confirmation of clinically atypical nevi does not establish the diagnosis of the FAMMM syndrome in any single individual under analysis. The histologic findings of an atypical nevus may be found in nevi of normal individuals. Ackerman (1988) believes that the histologic spectrum of AN extends into the histologic characteristics of normal nevi and the boundary between them is an arbitrary decision. He believes that "dysplastic naevus is not dysplastic because the term dysplasia has yet to be defined in an intelligible way; is not a syndrome because a single finding does not constitute a syndrome; and is not the commonest precursor of malignant melanoma because most melanomas arise de novo and not in preexisting melanocytic naevi." This view would appear to support the position of Piepkorn et al. (1989) who found clinically atypical nevi in the spouse controls and confirmed the clinical findings histologically. Thus, the security of histologic interpretation in a patient with AN is only absolute when it is negative for dysplasia; that is, if the clinically atypical nevus is normal histologically, then we are assured that it is a normal nevus and not an atypical nevus. A confirmed histologic presence of dysplastic nevi can only be interpreted as diagnostic when other clinical cutaneous phenotypic characteristics of the FAMMM syndrome (i.e., two or more of the following: total number of nevi is greater than normal, the presence of more than one large AN, and the occurrence of malignant melanoma) are present not only in the patient but in first and second degree relatives.

Systemic Cancer and the FAMMM Syndrome

Within the many cancer-associated genodermatoses, a pervasive theme at the clinical descriptive level has been their extant tumor heterogeneity. Indeed, this has become the hallmark of the more than 50 cancer-associated genodermatoses (Lynch and Fusaro 1982). The newest member of the group, the FAMMM syndrome, is no exception. Certainly, the full spectrum of its tumor heterogeneity remains the subject of intensive investigation (Bergman et al. 1986; Eusebi and Cook 1986; Lynch et al. 1981, 1982a,b, 1983; Lynch and Fusaro 1982). It is axiomatic that if one focuses energy exclusively upon the study of malignant melanoma in the FAMMM, and ignores cancer of all anatomic sites, one will necessarily come to the conclusion that the FAMMM predisposes only to malignant melanoma. Historically, this has been the experience in cancer-associated genodermatoses and other hereditary cancer syndromes, with the result that tumor spectra of these disorders were greater than previously conceived.

There have been several in-depth investigative reports concerning the occurrences of systemic cancer(s) in patients and their relatives with the FAMMM syndrome. The first of these was our study of four FAMMM kindreds (Figs. 2 and 5–7; Lynch et al. 1980, 1981, 1982b, 1983) which showed not only an increased rate of CMM, but also a significant 5-fold increase ($p < 0.004$) of systemic cancers of variable anatomic sites such as intraocular melanoma, cancer of the breast, respiratory tract, gastrointestinal tract, and lymphatic system (Table 2; Lynch et al. 1983a). Multiple unusual and diverse cancers in individual pedigree members were found, such as:

(a) squamous cell carcinoma of the tonsil and separate primary CMM in a 28-year-old female who rarely drank alcohol or smoked cigarettes (Fig. 5; Lynch et al. 1983b, and

Table 2. Cancer table ($n = 42$ gene carriers). (From Lynch et al. 1983)

	No. of patients	Observed (%)	Expected (%) (age-adjusted)
CMM	21	50.0	—
Atypical nevi	23	54.8	—
No CMM or nevi	3	7.1	—
Lung	3	7.1	0.8 ($p < 0.02$)[a]
Pancreas	2	4.8	0.2 ($p < 0.02$)[a]
Breast	2	4.8	0.6 ($p < 0.04$)[a]
Prostate	1	2.4	—
Tonsil	1	2.4	—
Larynx	1	2.4	—
All non-CMM cancer (all sites)	9[b]	21.4	4.1 ($p < 0.004$)[a]

[a] Exact probability of X or more affected calculated using binomial expansion
[b] One patient had both lung and prostate cancer

(b) intraocular melanoma (Fig. 6) in a FAMMM pedigree from Leiden, the Netherlands, where one of the members not only had bilateral intraocular melanoma primaries, one year apart, but multiple AN and several primary CMMs (Lynch et al. 1981; Oosterhuis et al. 1981).

Bergman et al. (1990) investigated cancer of *all* anatomic sites in nine FAMMM kindreds which were ascertained in a clinic for pigmented lesions in the Netherlands. A significant excess of systemic cancer (particularly involving the gastrointestinal tract) was observed in three of these nine families. The remaining families showed normal expectations of cancer, based on Dutch incidence data, among FAMMM gene carriers and their first degree relatives. Interestingly, in these families, there was an excessive number of cancers of the gastrointestinal tract. Nine of 18 cancers involved the pancreas, while none was colorectal cancer. This contrasted with Dutch incidence data in which half of the gastrointestinal tract cancers were of the colorectum, while approximately 10% involved the pancreas. All of the pancreatic cancers were adenocarcinomas. The fact that three of these nine families showed a marked excess of systemic cancer, while the remaining families showed normal numbers of cancer among those with the FAMMM genotype and their first degree relatives, indicated significant heterogeneity among these families.

Studies of the FAMMM syndrome which claim to have demonstrated a negative history for systemic cancer excess have been deficient in their verification methodology. Kopf et al. (1986) reported no evidence for systemic cancer in patients with familial malignant melanoma. An analysis of the data showed the methodology to have been based on interview, physical examination, and questionnaire, which was restricted to the proband and his recall of family history. This study did not involve an analysis of other members of the family, therefore, it was not an in-depth genetic study and does not contribute to the understanding

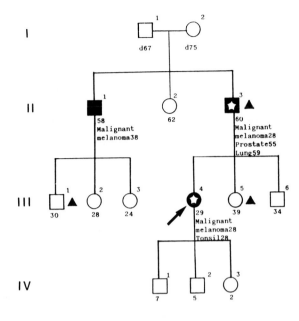

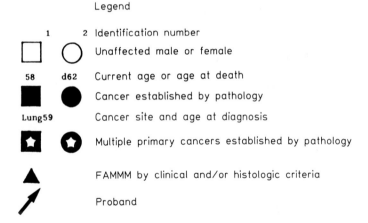

Legend

1	2	Identification number

□ ○ Unaffected male or female

58   d62   Current age or age at death

■ ● Cancer established by pathology

Lung59   Cancer site and age at diagnosis

★ ★ Multiple primary cancers established by pathology

▲ FAMMM by clinical and/or histologic criteria

↗ Proband

Fig. 5. Pedigree showing an unusual systemic cancer, tonsillar carcinoma in a young female. (From Lynch et al. 1983)

of hereditary malignant melanoma and its natural history, inclusive of systemic cancer association. Lynch et al. (1979) have shown in the past that restrictive genetic investigations which rely on limited recall of the proband give misleading data with respect to cancer occurrences in the kindred.

Greene et al. (1987) performed a prospective study of 14 kindreds at the NIH with hereditary CMM and the dysplastic nevus syndrome (DNS). They con-

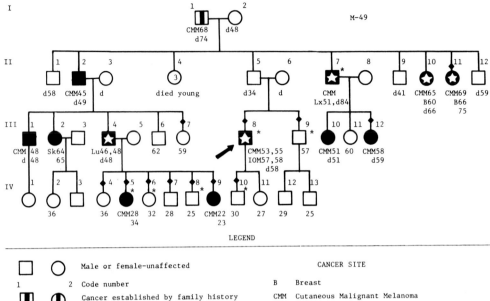

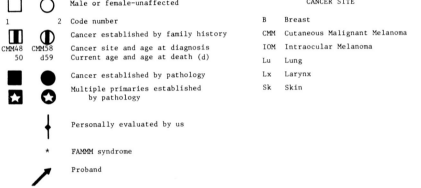

LEGEND

Fig. 6. Pedigree showing an unusual bilateral intraocular melanoma (IOM) in a member who had multiple cutaneous malignant melanomas (CMMs) and other tumors in obligate gene carriers. (From Lynch et al. 1981)

cluded that "no significant excess of nonmelanoma cancers was documented, suggesting that hereditary cutaneous malignant melanoma/dysplastic nevus syndrome are not pleiotropic for other tumor types." These conclusions were based on a negative finding which is weak in its statistical power, and both restrictive and biased in its patient selection. The study covers an approximate five-year period and is not adequate for the development of the phenotypic expression of systemic cancer which in hereditary cancer syndromes requires several generations for development of characteristics patterns. If one calculates the expression of systemic cancer with the use of only defined gene carriers (those with dysplastic nevi and/or malignant melanoma), their data show that there is a significant increase in the occurrence of gastrointestinal cancer ($p < 0.05$). Since these numbers were small, the authors considered them to be insufficient to

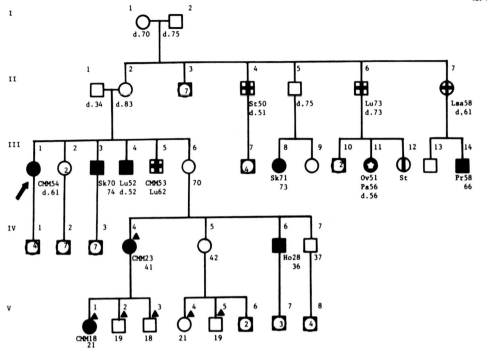

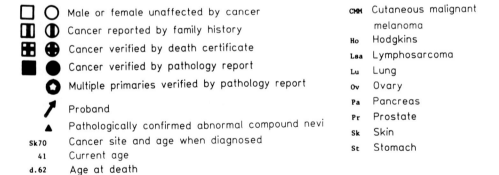

Fig. 7. Pedigree showing a female member (III-6) with no systemic or cutaneous phenotype and cancer-free at age 70 but by virtue of her position in the pedigree is a putative obligate gene carrier. Since this pedigree was published, individuals V-2 and V-3 have developed CMM. (From Lynch et al. 1980)

support the hypothesis of an excess of nonmelanotic cancer in the dysplastic nevus syndrome. It would be important to know in this study if the cancers were limited to only a few kindreds rather than all 14 kindreds, thereby verifying the concept of heterogeneity which appears to be common in cancer-associated genodermatoses, and increasing the significance of the cancer finding because of the smaller cohort size of the gene carriers.

Gene Linkage Studies and the FAMMM Syndrome

Appropriately, research has focused on chromosomal localization of the gene for DNS. Noteworthy was the report by Bale et al. (1989) which involved the study of 99 relatives and 26 spouses in six families who were predisposed to melanoma. Of these individuals, 34 had CMM, while 31 of these 34 showed histologic confirmation of DN. Twenty-four relatives showed dysplastic nevi (DN) alone. These findings indicated that the deleterious gene was on the distal part of the short arm of chromosome 1 (1p36) in a region between an anonymous DNA marker (D1S47) and the gene locus for pronatrodilatin (PND). The probe for D1S47 and PND showed lod scores of 3.62 and 3.09, respectively. The authors concluded that the odds were greater than 260 000 : 1 in support of linkage at this location.

However, vanHaeringen et al. (1989) performed linkage studies in six large Dutch DNS families. These investigators failed to find support for linkage between the loci for DNS and the Rhesus blood group on chromosome 1. They concluded that ". . . data from additional markers (DNF15S1, D1Z2, FUCA1, D1S17, D1S57, and PGM1) make it possible to exclude the DNS gene from the short arm of chromosome 1 in these Dutch families."

In collaboration with Mark Leppert and Ray White, we have also excluded linkage on the short arm of chromosome 1 in the investigation of two extended FAMMM kindreds. These findings will be the subject of a future report.

An explanation for these discrepant findings remains elusive. It is possible that heterogeneity among the American (Bale et al. 1989) and the Dutch (vanHaeringen et al. 1989) DNS kindreds could have contributed to some of these discrepancies. Variable expressivity and penetrance of the FAMMM gene must also be considered (Lynch et al. 1983a). In addition, there is an absence of any well-defined and accepted criteria for the minimal expression needed for a diagnosis of FAMMM in individual patients. Specifically, this is evidenced by the fact that a genotypically affected patient may have a complete absence of FAMMM moles (Lynch et al. 1983b) and yet express CMM. On the other hand, a patient may have neither DN, CMM, nor other systemic cancer, but be an obligate gene carrier by virtue of his or her position within the pedigree (Lynch et al. 1980).

Cytogenetics

Jaspers et al. (1987) carried out cytogenetic investigations on 25 individuals who were members of six DNS kindreds. Comparison was made between patients with DNS without a history of melanoma and their clinically normal relatives, as well as unrelated normal controls. These investigators indicated that normal frequencies of hyperdiploidy and spontaneous SCEs in fibroblasts from these individuals were present. Karyotypic studies were conducted on the relatives from one of these kindreds. Of interest was the finding that "... DNS had a normal constitutional karyotype. In lymphocytes or fibroblasts from five patients, however, increased frequencies of cells with random chromosomal rearrangements were observed. These abnormalities, mainly translocations and inversions, were not found in two of the patients' spouses and in six clinically normal relatives. In the fibroblast cultures, considerable clonal selection of cytogenetically abnormal cells occurred."

In collaboration with Avery Sandberg, we have studied cytogenetics from cultured lymphocytes, skin, and AN from two extended FAMMM kindreds. Findings showed significant chromosomal breakage and nonrandom translocations. These abnormalities were observed primarily in AN and normal skin fibroblasts (Lynch et al., in preparation). It will now be important to verify our cytogenetic findings in other well-documented FAMMM kindreds. It will be equally important to determine whether these cytogenetic findings might be capable of predicting differences in phenotypic expression of DN, CMM, and systemic cancer among FAMMM patients/families. This cytogenetic marker(s) should also be helpful in identifying individuals who are presumptive obligate gene carriers but who otherwise have not expressed any stigmata of the FAMMM phenotype. Its value will also extend to the identification of persons who have subtle phenotypic findings but who clinically may be considered either equivocal or unaffected. It will be imperative to follow such patients in order to determine whether CMM and cancers of extramelanotic sites occur in association with these cytogenetic aberrations. Finally, the cytogenetic marker(s) should also be evaluated in the following settings:

(a) patients with sporadic AN and/or CMM,
(b) kindreds with familial melanoma in the *absence* of FAMMM phenotypic features, and
(c) genetic counseling with special consideration toward the detection of the disorder in the fetus (amniocentesis) or at birth.

Conclusion

We have provided a clinicopathologic/genetic survey of the FAMMM syndrome so that its value as a model for genetic epidemiologic research might be more fully appreciated by our readership. Further research into markers correlating with

FAMMM's genotype, as in the case of cytogenetics, should facilitate these research objectives.

Acknowledgment. We are deeply grateful for the technical assistance of Diane Stanley.

References

Ackerman AB (1988) What naevus is dysplastic, a syndrome, and the commonest precursor of malignant melanoma? A riddle and an answer. Histopathology 13:241–256

Bale SJ, Dracopoli NC, Tucker MA, Clark WH, Fraser MC, Stanger BZ, Green P, Donis-Keller H, Housman DE, Greene MH (1989) Mapping the gene for hereditary cutaneous malignant melanoma-dysplastic nevus to chromosome 1p. N Engl J Med 320:1367–1372

Bergman W, Palan A, Went LN (1986) Clinical and genetic studies in six Dutch kindreds with the dysplastic naevus syndrome. Ann Human Genet 50:249–258

Bergman W, Watson P, Jong J de, Lynch HT, Fusaro RM (1990) Systemic cancer and the FAMMM syndrome. Br J Cancer 61:932–936

Bondi EE, Clark WH, Elder D, Guerry D, Greene MH (1981) Topical chemotherapy of dysplastic melanocytic nevi with 5% fluorouracil. Arch Dermatol 117:89

Cawley EP (1952) Genetic aspects of malignant melanoma. Arch Derm Syph 65:440

Clark WH, Reimer RR, Greene M, Ainsworth AM, Mastrangelo MJ (1978) Origin of familial malignant melanoma from heritable melanocytic lesions: the B-K mole syndrome. Arch Dermatol 114:732–738

Crombie IK (1979) Racial differences in melanoma incidence. Cancer 40:185–193

Duggleby WF, Stoll H, Priore RL, Greenwald P, Saxon G (1981) A genetic analysis of melanoma — polygenic inheritance as a threshold trait. Am J Epidemiol 114:63–72

Editorial (1986) Familial moles and malignant melanoma in The Netherlands. Lancet ii:614

Elder DE, Goldman LI, Goldman SC, Greene MH, Clark WH (1980) Dysplastic nevus syndrome: a phenotypic association of sporadic cutaneous melanoma. Cancer 46:1787

Eusebi V, Cook MG (1986) Melanocytic dysplasia and internal malignancy. Clin Exp Dermatol 11: 84–86

Green A, Siskind V (1983) Geographical distribution of cutaneous melanoma in Queensland. Med J Aust 30:407–410

Greene MH, Tucker MA, Clark WH, Kraemer KH, Elder DE, Fraser MC (1987) Hereditary melanoma and the dysplastic nevus syndrome: the risk of cancers other than melanoma. J Am Acad Dermatol 16:792–797

Haeringen A van, Bergman W, Nelen MR, Koou-Meijs E van der, Hendrikse I, Wijnen JT, Meera Khan P, Klasen EC, Frants RR (1989) Exclusion of the dysplastic nevus syndrome (DNS) locus from the short arm of chromosome 1 by linkage studies in Dutch families. Genomics 5:61–64

Jaspers NGJ, Roza-deJongh EJM, Donselaar IG, Velzen-Tillemans JTM van, Hemel JO van, Rumke P, vanderKamp AWM (1987) Sister chromatid exchanges, hyperdiploidy, and chromosomal rearrangements studied in cells from melanoma-prone individuals belonging to families with the dysplastic nevus syndrome. Cancer Genet Cytogenet 24:33–43

Kopf AW, Hellman LJ, Rogers GS, Gross DF, Rigel DS, Friedman RJ, Levenstein M, Brown J, Golomb FM, Roses DF, Gumport SL, Mintzis MM (1986) Familial malignant melanoma. JAMA 256:1915–1919

Kopf AW, Friedman RJ, Rigesl DS (1990) Atypical mole syndrome. J Am Acad Dermatol 22:117–118

Lynch HT, Fusaro RM (1982) Genodermatoses and cancer. In: Lynch HT, Fusaro RM (eds) Cancer-associated genodermatoses. Reinhold, New York, pp 1–35

Lynch HT, Fusaro RM (1986) Hereditary malignant melanoma: a unifying etiologic hypothesis. Cancer Genet Cytogenet 20:301–304

Lynch HT, Krush AJ (1968) Heredity and malignant melanoma: implications for cancer detection. Can Med Assoc J 99:17–21

Lynch HT, Frichot BC, Lynch JF (1978) Familial atypical multiple mole melanoma syndrome. J Med Genet 15:352

Lynch HT, Follett KL, Lynch PM, Albano WA, Mailliard JA, Pierson RL (1979) Family history in an oncology clinic: implications for cancer genetics. JAMA 242:1268–1272

Lynch HT, Fusaro RM, Pester J, Lynch J (1980) Familial atypical multiple mole melanoma (FAMMM) syndrome: genetic heterogeneity and malignant melanoma. Br J Cancer 42:58–70

Lynch HT, Fusaro RM, Pester J, Oosterhuis JA, Went LN, Rumke P, Neering H, Lynch JF (1981) Tumor spectrum in the FAMMM syndrome. Br J Cancer 44:553 560

Lynch HT, Fusaro RM, Pester JA (1982a) Genetic heterogeneity and malignant melanoma. In: Lynch HT, Fusaro RM (eds) Cancer-associated genodermatoses. Reinhold, New York, pp 394–439

Lynch HT, Fusaro RM, Kimberling WJ, Lynch JF (1983a) Familial atypical multiple mole melanoma (FAMMM) syndrome: segregation analysis. J Med Genet 20:342–344

Lynch HT, Fusaro RM, Pester J, Albano WA, Lynch JF (1983b) Phenotypic variation in the familial atypical multiple mole melanoma syndrome (FAMMM). J Med Genet 20:25–29

Lynch HT, Fusaro RM, Kimberling WJ, Lynch JF (1985) The cutaneous evolution of nevi in a patient with familial atypical multiple mole melanoma syndrome. Pediatr Dermatol 2:289–293

Magnus K (1987) Epidemiology of malignant melanoma of the skin. In: U Veronesi, N Cascinelli, M Santinami (eds) (1987) Cutaneous melanoma. Academic Press, New York, pp 1–13

Norris W (1820) A case of fungoid disease. Edin Med Surg J 16:562

Oosterhuis JA, Went LN, Lynch HT (1981) Primary choroidal and cutaneous melanomas, bilateral choroidal melanomas, and familial occurrence of melanomas. Br J Ophthalmol 66:230–233

Piepkorn M, Meyer LJ, Goldgar D, Seuchter SA, Cannon-Albright LA, Skolnick MH, Zone JJ (1989) The dysplastic melanocytic nevus: a prevalent lesion that correlates poorly with clinical phenotype. J Am Acad Dermatol 20:407–415

Roser M, Bohm A, Oldigs M, Weichenthal M, Reimers U, Schmidt-Preuss U, Breitbart EW, Rudiger HW (1989) Ultraviolet-induced formation of micronuclei and sister chromatid exchange in cultured fibroblasts of patients with cutaneous malignant melanoma. Cancer Genet Cytogenet 41:129–137

Steijlen PM, Bergman W, Hermans J, Scheffer E, van Vloten WA, Ruiter DJ (1988) The efficacy of histopathological criteria required for diagnosing dysplastic naevi. Histopathology 12:289–298

III. Computer Applications

Computer Simulation Methods
in Human Linkage Analysis*

J. OTT

Introduction

Computer simulation (Monte Carlo) methods based on pseudo-random numbers
are used to solve certain problems for which analytical solutions are either too
complex or impractical. Many processes in real life crucially depend on initial
conditions and are so complex that analytical solutions are out of the question.
Simulating such processes on the computer often yields useful solutions. For
example, transportation departments in large cities routinely simulate street
traffic to analyze the causes of traffic congestion or to predict the effects of street
closures.

   Typically, computer simulation methods furnish approximate solutions for
which the degree of accuracy can generally be calculated by statistical methods.
If analytical solutions to a problem are possible, they are usually preferable to
Monte Carlo solutions because the analytic formulas may reveal dependencies
among variables and other structural properties of the problem. Such information is much more difficult to obtain from Monte Carlo methods, since it may be
necessary to repeat the simulation for many different sets of parameter values.

   In human genetics, unknown properties of analysis methods have often
been investigated by computer simulation. For example, it has been shown that
accurate formulation of ascertainment correction in segregation analyses is in
practice not very useful because the mode of ascertainment is often not exactly
known and even small deviations between assumed and true mode of ascertainment can lead to large biases (Greenberg 1986). Early proposals to use
simulation methods as analysis tools (Ott 1974, 1979) have only in recent years
been pursued further. Below, areas in human linkage analysis are identified
where computer simulation methods are currently employed (Ott 1989). These
methods are of particular relevance to the analysis of complex traits such as
cancers and psychiatric disorders.

* This work was supported by grants from the National Institutes of Mental Health (MH44292), the
  Muscular Dystrophy Foundation, and the W.M. Keck Foundation

Columbia University, Box 58, Department of Genetics, 722 West 168th Street, New York, NY 10032,
USA

H.T. Lynch and P. Tautu (Eds.)
Recent Progress
in the Genetic Epidemiology of Cancer
© Springer-Verlag Berlin Heidelberg 1991

Expected Lod Score

Each family type (e.g., a phase-unknown double-backcross mating with four offspring) contains a certain amount of "information" for linkage analysis, where this information content may be measured in several ways. The measure most commonly used in linkage analysis is the expected lod score, $E[Z(\Theta)]$ (Ott 1985), where $Z(\Theta)$ is the lod score at a given recombination fraction, Θ. The expected lod score is calculated analytically by evaluating all possible genotype configurations, g, in the family structure in question, and by computing the weighted average, $E[Z(\Theta)] = \Sigma_g P(g;\Theta)Z_g(\Theta)$, where $P(g;\Theta)$ is the probability of occurrence of genotype configuration g, and $Z_g(\Theta)$ is the lod score obtained for g. In practice, another way to measure information is to calculate the probability that the maximum lod score exceeds a certain fixed value, but such calculations are not considered here.

For complicated family structures, the number of genotype configurations is so large that their enumeration is virtually impossible. Then, the expected lod score may be approximated by computer simulation as follows. Consider a family pedigree segregating for both a disease gene and a genetic marker linked to it. With given allele frequencies at the disease and marker loci, one randomly assigns genotypes to the founders according to Hardy-Weinberg equilibrium and then simulates the segregation of disease and marker alleles down through the pedigree according to mendelian laws. The disease genotypes generated are now used to randomly determine disease phenotypes with the appropriate probabilities (penetrances at the disease locus). A linkage analysis is then carried out in the same manner as it would be performed with real data, and the lod score Z_1 is recorded. This completes the first replicate of the simulation. The process is then repeated with new random genotype assignments, leading to a lod score Z_i for the i-th replicate. The arithmetic mean of the lod scores Z_i over replicates then approximates the true expected lod score for the given family structure.

Predicting Genotypes or Risks Given Disease Phenotypes

The computer simulation described above is relatively easy to carry out. The resulting expected lod score represents a theoretical measure of the information content in the family structure considered. In practice, one is often more interested in the information content of families in which disease phenotypes are already known, before marker typing is carried out. In other words, one wishes to compute the conditional expected lod score, given observed phenotypes. Such calculations are much more complex, and the following approaches have been taken.

Boehnke (1986) assumed known disease genotypes for each family member, that is, he considered the problem of randomly selecting marker genotypes given disease genotypes. This problem is relatively easy to solve, and Boehnke (1986) implemented his solution in a computer program, SIMLINK, which is, due to the requirement of known disease genotypes, particularly applicable to dominantly inherited diseases. It has been used by many researchers to compute the expected lod score that one is likely to obtain from the available family data, given observed disease phenotypes and a hypothetical marker locus with recombination fraction, Θ, between marker and disease locus. Of course, the expected lod score depends on what is assumed on the distance between marker and disease, small values of Θ yielding higher expected lod scores than loose linkage. We usually postulate a marker with four equally frequent alleles, at $\Theta = 0.02$ to 0.5 from the disease locus.

An extension of Boehnke's (1986) approach to partially reduced penetrance was developed by Sandkuyl and Ott (1989), who allow for incomplete penetrance in individuals without children. Specifically, they approximated the conditional risk distribution (given disease phenotypes) for a proband (counselee) in genetic counseling, before marker typing is carried out. For example, such a conditional distribution determines with what probability a risk of carrying the disease gene will be smaller than 10% or larger than 90%, when marker typing is carried out. In families with missing key individuals, or when the marker locus has low polymorphism, one may have only a small chance of providing a meaningful risk.

Ploughman and Boehnke (1989) further extended calculations of conditional expected lod scores by allowing for incomplete penetrance at the disease locus, and they implemented their results in the SIMLINK program. This means that disease genotypes no longer have to be known.

A very general simulation method was developed by Ott (1989), in which marker genotypes are simulated recursively in such a way that the probability of the marker genotype of the i-th individual is calculated, given the disease phenotypes of all individual and the marker genotypes of the i-1 individuals already generated. Consequently, this approach allows for partial marker typing in some individuals and may be used, for example, to determine which individual should be typed next for a maximum expected lod score, given the results of previously typed family members. It has been implemented in a computer program, SLINK (Dr. Daniel Weeks, in preparation), which is a modified version of the LINKAGE programs (Lathrop et al. 1984). The SLINK program allows for any genetic model that can be handled by the LINKAGE programs.

Evaluating the Significance of a Maximum Lod Score

In a linkage study, the observed maximum lod score, Z_{obs}, is taken as a measure for the evidence for linkage, and when Z_{obs} exceeds the value 3, linkage is considered proven, that is, the test for linkage is taken to be significant. The critical maximum lod score of 3 was originally chosen (Morton 1955) for good power and low type I error (p-value) in sequential tests with a number of small families. In likelihood ratio tests as generally carried out today, the p-value associated with an observed maximum lod score is not generally known. Statistical considerations show that a critical maximum lod score of 3 leads to a different type I error depending on the family types investigated. For example, for 10 phase-unknown double-backcross families, it is equal to 0.001 when each family has two offspring and equal to 0.00003 when each family has three offspring (Table 3.11 in Ott 1985). This situation is comparable to carrying out chi-square tests with different degrees of freedom, but all one knows is the resulting chi-square value while the number of degrees of freedom is unknown. Fortunately, computer simulation methods can provide approximations to the p-value associated with the maximum lod score observed in a given study.

The p-value (empirical significance level) associated with a critical maximum lod score is defined as the probability, given absence of linkage ($\Theta = 0.5$), that the lod score exceeds that critical limit. Therefore, when a linkage study has been carried out leading to an observed maximum lod score, Z_{obs}, the simulation methods outlined in the previous section may be employed. Assuming absence of linkage and thus independence of marker genotypes and disease phenotypes, one simply has to generate genotypes at the marker locus and analyze each replicate in the same manner as the real linkage analysis was carried out. For each replicate, it is determined whether the maximum lod score it furnished exceeds Z_{obs}. The p-value is then approximated by the proportion of replicates in which the maximum lod score is larger than Z_{obs}.

In linkage analyses of complex traits such as cancer and psychiatric traits, one is generally unsure of the mode of inheritance and perhaps also of the genetically relevant diagnostic scheme. Researchers often try to overcome such problems by trying out various genetic models and diagnostic schemes (e.g., narrow, medium and broad disease definition). Since the lod score reported is the overall maximum lod score, under whatever assumed mode of inheritance and diagnostic scheme it occurred, this practice amounts to maximizing the lod score not only over recombination fractions but also over genetic models and diagnostic schemes. The resulting maximum lod score, thus, has many more "degrees of freedom" than under a fixed genetic model and diagnostic scheme. In other words, such a maximum lod score is inflated when compared with a maximum lod score obtained under regular conditions. To assess the significance of a lod score maximized over genetic models and diagnostic schemes, computed simulation may be used as described in the previous paragraph, that is, marker genotypes are generated and each replicate is analyzed and the lod score maximized as it was done in the real study.

An example of such a situation is a recent linkage analysis for schizophrenia versus chromosome 5 markers (Sherrington et al. 1988) in which the lod score was maximized over three diagnostic schemes and penetrance values ranging from 0.5 through 1. The resulting maximum lod score was equal to 6.5. A computer simulation was then carried out as outlined above to approximately simulate the analysis of Sherrington et al. (1988). Under absence of linkage, in 2000 replicates, only one furnished a lod score exceeding 3 (Ott et al. 1989) so that the p-value associated with a lod score maximized over diagnostic schemes and penetrances is approximated by $1/2000 = 0.0005$. None of the 2000 replicates yielded a maximum lod score higher than 6.5. Therefore, the p-value in the study of Sherrington et al. (1988) is estimated as 0, with a 95%-confidence interval for the true p-value ranging from 0 through 0.0015. The results of these authors are, thus, still significant. That their lod score was inflated can be seen when one counts the number of replicates with a lod score exceeding 2. For a fixed diagnostic scheme and penetrance value, there were usually only two or three replicates with maximum lod scores exceeding 2, but when the lod score was maximized over diagnostic schemes and penetrances, the maximum lod score exceeded the value 2 in 11 out of the 2000 replicates.

That the practice of maximizing lod scores over model parameters inflates the lod score was also shown in another computer simulation analysis (Clerget-Darpoux et al. 1990). Also, to work more efficiently with extreme values which are infrequently observed, the generated distribution of maximum lod scores can be fitted to suitable parametric distributions, which will permit "deflating" the maximum lod scores obtained under nonstandard conditions to better inter-pretable values (Ott et al. 1990).

Acknowledgment. Helpful comments by Dr. Daniel Weeks greatly improved an earlier version of the manuscript and are gratefully acknowledged.

References

Boehnke, M (1986) Estimating the power of a proposed linkage study: a practical computer simulation approach. Am J Hum Genet 39:513–527

Clerget-Darpoux F, Babron M-C, Bonaïti-Pellié C (1990) Assessing the effect of multiple linkage tests in complex diseases. Genet Epidemiol 7(4):245–253

Greenberg DA (1986) The effect of proband designation on segregation analysis. Am J Hum Genet 39:329–339

Lathrop GM, Lalouel JM, Julier C, Ott J (1984) Strategies for multilocus linkage analysis in humans. Proc Natl Acad Sci USA 81:3443–3446

Morton NE (1955) Sequential tests for the detection of linkage. Am J Hum Gen 7:277–318

Ott J (1974) Computer simulation in human linkage analysis (abstract). Am J Hum Genet 26:64A

Ott J (1979) Maximum likelihood estimation by counting methods under polygenic and mixed models in human pedigrees. Am J Hum Genet 31:161–175

Ott J (1985) Analysis of human genetic linkage. Johns Hopkins University Press, Baltimore

Ott J (1989) Computer-simulation methods in human linkage analysis. Proc Natl Acad Sci USA 86:4175–4178

Ott J, Lehner T, Squires-Wheeler E, Kaufmann C (1989) Linkage analysis – potential problems introduced by the pratice of maximizing the lod score over a wide range of parameters including disease classification (unpublished abstracts of First World Congress of Psychiatric Genetics, Cambridge, England)

Ploughman LM, Boehnke M (1989) Estimating the power of a proposed linkage study for a complex genetic trait. Am J Hum Genet 44:543–551

Sandkuyl LA, Ott J (1989) Determining informativity of marker typing for genetic counseling in a pedigree. Hum Genet 82:159–162

Sherrington R, Brynjolfsson J, Petursson H, Potter M, Dudleston K, Barraclough B, Wasmuth J, Dobbs M, Gurling H (1988) Localization of a susceptibility locus for schizophrenia on chromosome 5. Nature 336:164–167

Weeks D, Lehner T, Squares-Wheeler E, Kaufmann C, Ott J (1990) Measuring the inflation of the lod score due to its maximization over model parameter values in human linkage analysis. Genet Epidemiol 7(4):237–243

Computer Programs for Linkage Analysis*

J. OTT

Introduction

The main goal of linkage analysis is the estimation of the recombination fraction(s) between two (two-point analysis) or more loci (multipoint analysis). Only in very simple cases is it possible to obtain such estimates with pencil and paper. Usually, the calculations involved are so complex that a computer program has to be employed. Below, many of the frequently used programs are briefly described, although the list is by no means complete. Notice that programs for computer simulation are discussed in another section of this report. Also, programs for nonparametric linkage analysis (e.g., affected sib-pair methods) are not discussed in this outline.

In linkage analysis, parameter estimation is generally carried out by the maximum likelihood method. Linkage programs in principle calculate the likelihood of family data, that is, the probability of occurrence of the observed phenotypes. As the likelihood depends on the mode of inheritance (which may be specified through penetrances), on gene frequencies, recombination fractions, etc., values for these parameters have to be furnished by the user. Most programs can iteratively maximize the likelihood, either over recombination fractions only or over other parameter values as well. In multipoint calculations, probabilities of haplotypes (gametes) produced by a parent are generally calculated under the assumption that recombinations in the different intervals occur independently of each other (absence of interference). This assumption has been criticized for being unrealistic but its effect on gene mapping has not been thoroughly investigated.

Most of the linkage programs are available for various computer types, as well as for IBM microcomputers. Porting them to the Macintosh has proved somewhat difficult since the code must be broken down into small 32KB blocks. Interested people should contact Dr. Weeks.

As a means of quickly disseminating information to linkage analysts, I am distributing a Linkage Newsletter which is mailed out about twice a year free of

* This work was supported by grants from the National Institutes of Mental Health (MH44292), the Muscular Dystrophy Foundation, and the W.M. Keck Foundation

Columbia University, Box 58, Department of Genetics, 722 West 168th Street, New York NY 10032, USA

H.T. Lynch and P. Tautu (Eds.)
Recent Progress
in the Genetic Epidemiology of Cancer
© Springer-Verlag Berlin Heidelberg 1991

charge. It contains information on programs distributed by me and by other researchers, questions and contributions from readers, announcements of linkage courses, etc. To subscribe, please write to me.

The LIPED Program

LIPED (for likelihood in pedigrees) was the first generally available computer program for linkage analysis of simple and complex pedigrees (Ott 1976). It has been employed successfully in many linkage analyses and is still widely used, although it is limited to jointly analyzing no more than two loci. LIPED is written in Fortran and has been ported to various computers. I am currently supporting only the PC version of it.

The major advantages of the LIPED program are its dependability and the fact that it carries out many checks for consistency of the input data. Like many other programs, it recursively traverses pedigrees and calculates the likelihood by the Elston-Stewart algorithm (Elston and Stewart 1971). Marriage and consanguinity loops are handled by conditioning on the genotypes of one or more family members (Lange and Elston 1975). LIPED can only traverse a pedigree from the bottom up. Therefore, when two parents themselves both have parents (four grandparents) in the pedigree, conditioning on the genotypes of one of the two parents is required. This requirement is not present in newer linkage programs.

LIPED has options for calculating lod score tables for male and female recombination fractions. Also, it provides flexible age-of-onset curves (e.g., in disease loci with age-dependent penetrance).

The PAP Program

The PAP program was developed in Salt Lake City (Hasstedt and Cartwright 1981) and extends linkage analysis to more than two loci. Presently it can analyze up to four loci jointly. It is being used by many researchers. For details, the reader is referred to the original description of it.

The LINKAGE Programs

These programs form a package of several linkage programs (Lathrop et al. 1984) which carry out two-point and multipoint calculations in general pedigrees. The three main analysis programs are MLINK (lod score and risk calculation), LINKMAP (likelihood of one locus versus a map of loci), and ILINK (iterative parameter estimation). They are written in Pascal (Turbo Pascal on IBM microcomputers). In the ILINK program, parameters are estimated by a particular method of numerical maximization of the likelihood (Lalouel 1979).

Likelihood calculations are carried out by the Elston-Stewart algorithm, traversing pedigrees in the up or down direction. Loops are handled as in the LIPED program. A sex difference in the recombination fraction is parametrized by (1) male recombination fraction, and (2) female-to-male map distance ratio. For a lod score table of male versus female recombination fractions, transformation of these two parameters into male and female recombination fractions is required and may be carried out with one of the Linkage Utility programs available from me. Except for three-point analysis, the LINKAGE programs assume absence of interference.

The LINKAGE programs require good computer resources, particularly when many loci are analyzed jointly. On IBM microcomputers, no more than a total of six loci can be analyzed at once and, depending on the number of individuals and the number of alleles at the loci, the maximum number of loci that can be handled may be less than six.

For gene mapping, a specialized version of the LINKAGE programs is available (Lathrop and Lalouel 1988) which is directed to analyzing the CEPH reference pedigrees (three generations, two parents, at most four grandparents). Only codominant loci may be used, but many more loci than in the general LINKAGE programs can be analyzed jointly.

The LINKAGE programs are available from Dr. Mark Lathrop in Paris; the PC versions are also available from me.

The MAPMAKER Program

MAPMAKER (Lander et al. 1987) is specialized for analyzing the CEPH reference type families and mapping genetic marker loci. It is thus restricted to codominant loci. MAPMAKER is written in the C language. Several features set this program apart from other linkage programs. For example, it is "user-friendly", which is not generally the case for linkage programs.

In MAPMAKER, the special algorithm employed for calculating the likelihood depends more on the number of individuals in a pedigree than on the number of loci. This is one of the reasons why MAPMAKER is restricted to analyzing simple family types, but the advantage of this scheme is that a large number of loci may be analyzed jointly. For the estimation of recombination fractions, the likelihood is maximized by the EM algorithm.

The CRI-MAP Program

The CRI-MAP program was developed by Dr. P. Green, formerly at Collaborative Research, Inc., for rapid map construction using CEPH pedigrees and codominant loci. It has recently been extended to work on more general pedigrees and simple dominant systems (Goldgar et al. 1989). Information from untyped individuals at a given locus is incorporated in the analysis only when their genotypes at that locus can be inferred unequivocally.

The MENDEL Program

The capabilities of the MENDEL program (Lange et al. 1988) are comparable to those of the LINKAGE programs. The Fortran program MENDEL is part of the Programs for Pedigree Analysis package, which is available from its authors. It provides routines for special tasks (e.g., risk calculation, heterogeneity).

Consanguinity and marriage loops are handled differently than in LIPED and in the LINKAGE programs. Basically, all the information on family members outside of a loop is "condensed" onto individuals constituting the loop, and the loop is then analyzed unbroken. In some cases, this results in much faster analysis of pedigrees with a loop. On the other hand, the MENDEL program tends to require more memory than the LINKAGE programs for the analysis of the same problem.

Other Computer Programs

The LINKAGE programs mentioned above carry out likelihood calculations for family pedigree data. Their results are often reported in terms of lod scores (two-point or multipoint) or location scores. These, in turn, may then form the basis for other calculations which can be carried out by programs discussed below. Also mentioned below are two programs for data management.

The HOMOG programs (Ott 1985) address the problem of disease hete- rogeneity. They calculate likelihoods under the assumption of a mixture of families, where in different families the disease gene may be linked to different markers. In the simplest case, two family types are assumed, one with linkage to a marker or a map of markers, and one without linkage. Input to these programs are lod scores obtained from a linkage analysis.

The MAP program (Morton and Andrews 1989) combines two-point lod scores into multipoint lod scores for various loci under the assumption that the two-point lods are independent of each other.

A collection of Linkage Utility programs are available from me for various special tasks. For example, the MAPFUN program converts recombination fractions into map distances and vice versa using six mapping functions. For a given male recombination fraction and a mapping function, the SEXDIF pro- gram converts a female recombination fraction into the corresponding female- to-male map distance ratio and vice versa.

The dGENE program (Lange et al. 1988) is a database program, which has been developed to enter, manipulate, and retrieve family data and locus data. It is written in dBASE and is primarily used in conjunction with the MENDEL program but has recently been generalized by Dr. Daniel Weeks to produce files in the format required by the LINKAGE programs. Another data management program, LINKSYS, has been developed by John Attwood at University College, London. It is written in Turbo Pascal and provides data storage and retrieval for the LIPED and LINKAGE programs.

References

Elston RC, Stewart J (1971) A general model for the analysis of pedigree data. Hum Hered 21:523–542

Goldgar DE, Green P, Parry DM, Mulvihill JJ (1989) Multipoint linkage analysis in Neurofibromatosis type I: an international collaboration. Am J Hum Genet 44:6–12

Hasstedt SJ, Cartwright PE (1981) PAP – Pedigree Analysis Package, University of Utah, Department of Medical Biophysics and Computing, Technical Report No. 13. Salt Lake City, Utah

Lalouel JM (1979) GEMINI – a computer program for optimization of general nonlinear functions. University of Utah, Department of Medical Biophysics and Computing, Technical Report No. 14. Salt Lake City, Utah

Lander ES, Green P, Abrahamson J, Barlow A, Daly MJ, Lincoln SE, Newburg L (1987) MAPMAKER: an interactive computer package for constructing primary genetic linkage maps of experimental and natural populations. Genomics 1:174–181

Lange K, Elston RC (1975) Extensions to pedigree analysis. I. Likelihood calculations for simple and complex pedigrees. Hum Hered 25:95–105

Lange K, Weeks D, Boehnke M (1988) Programs for pedigree analysis: MENDEL, FISHER, and dGENE. Genet Epidemiol 5:471–472

Lathrop GM, Lalouel J-M (1988) Efficient computations in multilocus linkage analysis. Am J Hum Genet 42:498–505

Lathrop GM, Lalouel JM, Julier C, Ott J (1984) Strategies for multilocus linkage analysis in humans. Proc Natl Acad Sci USA 81:3443–3446

Morton NE, Andrews V (1989) MAP, an expert system for multiple pairwise linkage analysis. Ann Hum Genet 53:263–269

Ott J (1976) A computer program for linkage analysis of general human pedigrees. Am J Hum Genet 28:528–529

Ott J (1985) Analysis of human genetic linkage. Johns Hopkins University Press, Baltimore

A Comprehensive Pedigree Analysis Tool: FAP (Family Analysis Package)*

M. Neugebauer and M.P. Baur

Introduction

A major problem in genetic epidemiology is the analysis of human pedigrees. The purpose of this analysis may be to determine the mode of inheritance of a disease, to test linkage, or to calculate risk factors for an individual, when it is known that a genetic disease is segregating within a family. Pedigree analysis unifies the approach to all three of these problems.

The 9th International HLA Workshop 1984 initiated the need for a program which is able to handle multilocus pedigree data of any size. The Family Analysis Package (FAP) has been developed to estimate the population frequencies (Albert et al. 1984). Since then, new features have been added to the FAP in order to get a comprehensive pedigree analysis tool.

Given a genetic model, the FAP calculates the likelihood for a pedigree with multilocus data. This likelihood calculation can be used for different analysis strategies, such as:

— "Haplotyping of families"
— Estimation of n-locus-haplotype frequencies (i.e., gene frequencies, two-locus-linkage disequilibria, etc.)
— Estimation of penetrance values
— n-locus-linkage analysis
— Maximum likelihood ordering in linkage groups
— Risk calculation for genetic counseling
— Risk calculation for paternity testing
— Risk calculation with different population codes in a pedigree

The genetic model can be freely defined including parameter values for:

— Phenotype-genotype relation
— Allele frequencies
— Two-locus-linkage disequilibria
— Recombination frequencies
— Penetrance values

* Supported by Deutsche Forschungsgemeinschaft DFG Ba 66015-3

Institut für Med. Statistik, Dokumentation, und Datenverarbeitung, Sigmund-Freud-Str. 25, W-5300 Bonn-Venusberg, FRG

H.T. Lynch and P. Tautu (Eds.)
Recent Progress
in the Genetic Epidemiology of Cancer
© Springer-Verlag Berlin Heidelberg 1991

— Age correction for penetrance
— Quantitative penetrance function
— X-chromosomal inheritance, including pseudoautosomal inheritance
— Mutation

The program is able to analyze:

— Pedigrees with multiple recombinations
— Pedigrees with missing or partially missing phenotype data of some members
— Pedigrees with any kind of inbreeding

There are in general no restrictions to the number of loci, the pedigree structure, or the number of generations, except the available CPU time and the size of the main storage. FAP consists of a system of PL/1 routines. The program package uses only standard features of PL/1 (except two functions, which can easily be replaced, see Neugebauer 1990). Thus an implementation on any computer supporting the language PL/1 should be possible. There exists a version for IBM with operating system VM/CMS or MVS. This package is being made generally available.

Researchers who like to work with a more user-friendly menu driven interface to FAP can make use of the VM/CMS macro RUNFAP, which manages the FAP control parameters (see Fig. 1). For any other operating system this macro has to be rewritten. For further information see the technical report of FAP (Neugebauer 1990) or the user manual for FAP (Seuchter et al. 1990).

Methods

The likelihood of a pedigree is the probability P ("DATA"/MODEL), where MODEL is the definition of the genetic model and DATA are the phenotypes in the pedigree and the pedigree structure. The formula for the likelihood for a general pedigree was first given by Elston and Stewart (1971).

Likelihood Calculation

Likelihood Formula

Given the phenotype of an individual and a phenotype-genotype relation, it is possible to create all genotypes. So the likelihood is given as a sum over all genotypes of all individuals:

$$L = \sum_{k_1 \varepsilon G_1} \sum_{k_2 \varepsilon G_2} \cdots \sum_{k_{n_{ipi}} \varepsilon G_{n_{ipi}}} \prod_{i=1}^{n_{ipi}} \mathrm{Pen}(i,k_i) \prod_{\substack{i=1 \\ \mathrm{unrelated}}}^{n_{ipi}} f(k_i) \prod_{(k_{i_1}; k_{i_2}, k_{i_3})} \mathrm{trans}(k_{i_1}; k_{i_2}, k_{i_3})$$

FAP analysis possibilities: please select one	
0/blank	: No modification to the CONTROL file
1	: Haplotyping with a short output
1A	: Risk calculation
1B	: Paternity testing
2	: Haplotyping with a detailed output
3	: Estimation of haplotype frequencies
4	: Pairwise linkage analysis of all loci
5	: Pairwise linkage analysis with the 1. locus
6	: Order of all loci
7	: Order of the disease locus in a given marker map
8	: Estimation of recombination fraction (more than two loci)
9	: Loci ordering and estimation of recombination fraction (combination of 7 and 8)

Fig. 1. Main menu of FAP

$Pen(i,k_i)$: penetrance = probability of phenotype i under the condition of genotype k_i

$f(k_i)$: population frequency of genotype k_i for the founder individuals

Trans : transmission probability = mendelian ratios (1/2,1/4,1) and crossover frequencies

If n_i is the number of different possible genotypes for individual i, the likelihood is a sum over $m = n_1 \cdot n_2 \cdots n_{n_{ipi}}$ partial likelihoods:

$$L = \sum_m L \text{ (pedigree/genotype explanation)}$$

L(pedigree explanation) is the part of the likelihood from one pedigree explanation. A pedigree explanation is the assignment of only one genotype to each individual. So this assignment is one possible explanation of the pedigree with the phenotype data. If the total likelihood L is known, for each pedigree explanation a relative likelihood can be given:

$$L_{rel}(j) = \frac{L(j)}{\sum_{k=1}^{m} (L(k))}$$

(relative likelihood for explanation j)

In the same manner a relative likelihood for a genotype can be given, as a sum over all relative likelihoods of pedigree explanations, which contains the genotype:

$$L(\text{genotype} = g) = \sum_{g \in j} L_{rel}(j)$$

If we consider n-locus data, the term diplotype is used instead of genotype. The diplotype is the ordered tupel of paternal haplotype and maternal haplotype: diplotype = (paternal haplotype, maternal haplotype). And the haplotype is the set of alleles which is inherited on one chromosome. So in the following, the likelihood formula is explained for n-locus data. For each member of the pedigree

$i = 1 \cdots n_{ipi}$ a diplotype set with n_i diplotypes $(D_{i_1} \ldots D_{i_{n_i}})$ exists. From this one can give $m = n_1 \cdot n_2 \cdots n_{n_{ipi}}$ different possible pedigree-explanations with only one diplotype per individual. The summation over these m-explanations gives the likelihood of the whole pedigree:

$$L = \sum_{D_1=1}^{n_1} \cdots \sum_{D_{n_{ipi}}=1}^{n_{ipi}} \prod_{i=1}^{n_{ipi}} Pen(i,D_i) \prod_{\substack{i=1 \\ unrelated}}^{n_{ipi}} f(D_i) \prod_{\substack{(D_{i_1};D_{i_2},D_{i_3}) \\ related}} trans(D_{i_1}; D_{i_2}, D_{i_3})$$

$Pen(i,D_i)$: penetrance = probability of phenotype i under the condition of diplotype D_i

$f(D_i)$: population frequency of diplotype D_i for the founder individuals

Trans : transition probability = mendelian ratios $(1/2, 1/4, 1)$ and crossover frequencies

The program first calculates the haplotype frequencies (= diplotype frequencies) and then the likelihood of the various possibilities and sums up all likelihood values. For each explanation $j = 1...m$ the relative likelihood is computed

$$l_{rel}(j) = \frac{L(j)}{\sum_{k=1}^{m} (L(k))}$$

With these values each diplotype D_{i_k} of individual i has a relative likelihood:

$$L_{rel}(D_{i_k}) = \sum_{\substack{j=1 \\ D_{i_k} \, \varepsilon \, \text{Explanation j}}}^{m} L_{rel}(j)$$

This algorithm is used for haplotyping families. An example is given in the section "Haplotyping in Pedigrees", below.

Calculation of the Haplotype Frequencies

For unlinked loci the haplotype frequency is given by the product of the allele frequencies:

$f(a,b,c) = f(a)f(b)f(c)$

For linked loci the haplotype frequency calculation must take into account disequilibrium values $(\Delta(a,b))$. For n-locus haplotypes the frequency in the population is normally not known, so for these frequencies approximations must be made.

The program is only able to handle two-loci disequilibria $(\Delta(a,b))$. Here, the frequency of a two-loci haplotype is given by:

$f(a,b) = f(a)f(b) + \Delta(a,b)$

For multilocus haplotypes the frequency is approximated in the following way:

$$f(a,b) = f(a)f(b) + \Delta(a,b)$$
$$f(a,b,c) = f(c)f(a,b)$$
$$+ f(a) \Delta(b,c)$$
$$+ f(b) \Delta(a,c)$$
$$f(a,b,c,d) = f(d) f(a,b,c)$$
$$+ f(a,b) \Delta(c,d)$$
$$+ f(a,c) (\Delta(b,d)$$
$$+ f(b,c) \Delta(a,d)$$

for a n-loci haplotype f is given as follows:

$$f(a_1,...a_i,...,a_n) = f(a_1,...a_i,...,a_{n-1}) f(a_n)$$
$$+ \sum_{\substack{j=1 \\ i \neq j, i \neq n}}^{n-1} f(a_1,...,a_i,...,a_{n-2}) \Delta(a_j, a_n)$$

Calculation of the Penetrance

The penetrance is the probability of having a phenotype conditional on the genotype: penetrance = P(phenotype/genotype). This penetrance is defined for the genotypes of one locus and the phenotype belongs to the considered locus. For qualitative traits a penetrance value must be given for each phenotype and each genotype at the considered locus. The program expects the following penetrance values in matrix format for each phenotype:

Phenotype "PH"	allele$_1$	allele$_2$
allele 1	P_{11}	P_{12}
allele 2	P_{21}	P_{22}

$P_{ij} = P(\text{"PH"}/\text{allele}_i, \text{allele}_j)$ is the penetrance given the genotype "allele$_1$, allele$_2$" for the phenotype "PH".

Although this matrix is symmetric for most of the cases, it is possible to have different penetrance values for sex-dependent penetrance. The alleles given in the top row of the matrix are the alleles which were transmitted from the father, the alleles given in the column were transmitted from the mother: $P(\text{Ph}/\text{allele}_1, \text{allele}_2)$ is the penetrance having the phenotype PH, the alleles, with allele$_1$ inherited from the mother and allele$_2$ inherited from the father; $P(\text{PH}/\text{allele}_2, \text{allele}_1)$ is the corresponding penetrance, having the allele$_1$ from the father, allele$_2$ from the mother. For individuals which have no parents in the pedigree the mean of the two values is used.

For quantitative traits the penetrance must be calculated in an easy way from a quantitative phenotype. For this Gauss density is used:

$$\text{Pen}(\text{PH} / a_1, a_2) = \frac{1}{2\pi\sigma} \, e^{- \left(\frac{ph - ph_{a_1.a_2}}{\sigma_{a_1.a_2}} \right)^2}$$

For each genotype a mean value and a variance must be given.

Calculation of the Transmission Probabilities

The transmission probability trans($K_{i_1}/k_{i_2}, k_{i_3}$) is the probability that a child has the genotype k_{i_1} if the father has the genotype k_{i_2} and the mother has the genotype k_{i_3}. This is mainly determined by the mendelian ratios. If a parent is heterozygous the transmission probability is 1/2, while if the parent is homozygous the transmission probability is 1; so for both parents the probabilities are 1, 1/2 or 1 depending on the heterozygosity. For multilocus pedigrees the second factor for the transmission probability is the recombination fraction between two adjacent loci. With no interferences the "crossover function" for m-loci is given as follows:

$$C(\eta) = \prod_{j=1}^{m-1} \theta_j^{\eta_j} (1 - \theta_j)^{1-\eta}$$

η is a vector of dimension $n = m-1$; where η_j is 1, if a crossover occurred between locus j and locus j+1, η_j is 0 if there is no crossover between these loci. θ_j is the recombination fraction between locus j and locus j+1.

Estimation Procedures

As shown above a lot of parameters must be given to calculate the likelihood of a pedigree. Reversely a set of family data parameters can be estimated by maximizing the total likelihood. FAP can be used to estimate haplotype frequencies, which include allele frequencies and linkage-disequilibria values to estimate recombination fractions, and the program can be used to estimate penetrance values. FAP uses the iterative EM-algorithm (Estimation and Maximization); the likelihood and the relative likelihood values are calculated from the data set, new parameters are estimated by counting the relative likelihoods (for haplotypes, crossovers, or penetrance) and the likelihood is calculated again with these new estimated parameters. This is done iteratively and at the end (maximum number of iterations reached or increase of the total likelihood smaller than a certain value) the likelihood and the estimated parameters are given.

Estimation of Haplotype Freqeuncies

Family data can be used to estimate haplotype frequencies, allele frequencies, and linkage-disequilibria. By using family data for estimation of haplotype frequencies it is possible to get the phase for the diplotypes, and the estimation is done for gametes. For the estimation of haplotypes only the diplotypes of the unrelated individuals are used. The estimation gives as a result the estimated haplotype frequencies at each iteration and after the last iteration the allele frequencies and optional two-loci-linkage-disequilibria values. The results of an estimation can be used as input for a new analysis.

Linkage Analysis

The estimation of recombination fractions is called linkage analysis. This estimation of the recombination fraction between two loci is done without interference. The program is able to deal with all pairwise loci independently or a set of loci with a given order. This means one can analyze a set of families including three loci A-B-C and estimate the recombination fractions θ_{A-B} and θ_{B-C} or one can analyze the data for all pairwise loci independently (A-B and B-C). For the first kind of analysis the program gives a combined lod score and the estimated θ values; for the second kind of analysis the individual lod scores and θ values are calculated. The estimation can be done with the EM algorithm to get an optimal lod score, or a table of lod scores of a set of θ values can be calculated. All these analyses are possible with different θ values optional by sex.

Test for Different Loci Orders

By calculating likelihood values for different loci orders, a test for these orders can be performed. Optionally a trait can be moved through a given marker map, or all possible loci orders can be considered.

Data Structure for FAP

To run FAP, the program needs three input files with the following information:

PEDDATA Pedigree data: individual identification, mother and father identification, phenotype data, sex, disease status, etc.

GENSYS Description of the genetic systems: names of loci and alleles, linkage disequilibrium (two-point), paternal and maternal recombination fraction, mutation rate, order of loci, penetrance, etc.

CONTROL Parameters to control the different kinds of analyses: haplotyping of families, linkage analysis, estimation of haplotypes, penetrance, risk calculation, etc. In the second part the format of the pedigree data (PEDDATA) is described.

For a more detailed description see Seuchter et al. (1990).

Haplotyping in Pedigrees

The following example is of a 3-generation family with phenotype data for HLA loci A,C and B. The following program printout gives the pedigree phenotype data, all possible haplotype frequencies (calculated from the population frequencies), all formal genetic possible diplotypes for each individual, the most likely pedigree explanation, and all relative likelihoods for each diplotype of each individual. In this example with one locus there exists only one unique solution. Allele HLA A10 is divided in two split alleles HLA A25 and HLA A26.

crossover is marked with $\neq$; a crossover in a range of loci, which cannot be uniquely marked because of homozygosity is indicated by ':'.

Pedigree :		2			Family 1							
Fam	Ind :	Pat	Mat	Sex	Pop :	A	A	B	B	C	C :	
2	1 :			1	0 :	2	32	27	62	2	3 :	
2	2 :			2	0 :	10					:	
2	3 :	1	2	1	0 :	26	32	8	27	2	7 :	
2	4 :	1	2	2	0 :	25	32	18	27	2	5 :	
2	5 :	1	2	2	0 :	25	32	18	27	2	5 :	
2	6 :	1	2	1	0 :	25	32	8	27	2	5 :	
2	7 :			2	0 :	2	1	8		0	:	
2	8 :	6	7	1	0 :	25	1	8		5	:	
Used population code:												

***** Possible   A/   C — crossover *****
***** Possible   C/   B — crossover *****

Phenotype data for loci HLA A,C and B

For each individual of this pedigree up to 4 different diplotype explanations are possible, (for example of IND 1: (2,27,2/32,62,3), (2,62,2/32,27,3), (2,62,3/32,27,2), (2,27,3/32,62,2)). Thus theoretically $4^8 = 65536$ different pedigree explanations must be considered neglecting the formal genetic reduction.

Used population code:			0
Used haplotypes in pedigree (HFRC = 1)			
Haplotype			Frequency
A	C	B	
26	7	8	0.001760
25	5	18	0.001063
26	7	18	0.000460
25	5	8	1.0000E-12
2	3	27	0.001880
32	2	62	0.000352
2	3	62	0.017501
32	2	27	0.000987
2	0	8	0.000557
1	0	0	0.000331
2	0	0	0.001004
1	0	8	0.015766
26	5	8	1.0000E-12
25	7	18	0.003288
26	5	18	0.000226
25	7	8	0.001208
2	2	27	0.006265
32	3	62	0.002171
2	2	62	0.000611
32	3	27	0.000177

Approximated haplotype frequencies, used for likelihood calculation.

Most likely pedigree explanations					
-log10 (likelihood), (max) = 20.2305, (20.2305)					
Pedigree explanation Prel = 0.6332					
Ind	Pat	Mat	A	C	B
1			2	3	62
			32	2	27
2			26	7	8
			25	5	18
3	1	2	32	2	27
			26	7	8
4	1	2	32	2	27
			25	5	18
5	1	2	32	2	27
			25	5	18
6	1	2	32	2	27
			25	5	8
7			2	0	0
			1	0	8
8	6	7	25	5	8
			1	0	8
1. Pedigree explanation					

In individual 6 a crossover is marked between locus C and B.

Relative likelihoods of diplotypes						
Ind	Pat	Mat	A	C	B	rel. likelihood
1			2	3	62	1.000000
			32	2	27	
2			26	7	8	1.000000
			25	5	18	
3	1	2	32	2	27	1.000000
			26	7	8	
4	1	2	32	2	27	1.000000
			25	5	18	
5	1	2	32	2	27	1.000000
			25	5	18	
6	1	2	32	2	27	1.000000
			25	5	8	
7			2	0	0	0.638286
			1	0	8	
			2	0	8	0.354286
			1	0	8	
			2	0	8	0.007428
			1	0	0	
8	6	7	25	5	8	0.987534
			1	0	8	
			25	5	8	0.012466
			1	0	0	
Used CPU time: 2.20						

Discussion

FAP is a program package which was mainly designed for haplotyping of families and was enlarged for general likelihood calculations in pedigrees. A comparison with other programs like LIPED or LINKAGE during the Genetic Analysis Workshop III (MacCluer 1985) showed good results for FAP. In contrast to other analysis programs FAP is the only one with the following features:

— Analysis of loci with in principle unlimited number of alleles (no recording necessary)
— Analysis of pedigrees with inbreeding (no recording necessary)
— Different allele frequencies for different populations within a pedigree
— Use of linkage disequilibria
— Estimation of haplotype frequencies

Some of these features may be interesting in special fields like population genetics or risk calculation.

References

Albert ED, Baur MP, Mayr WR (eds) (1984) Histocompatibility testing 1984. Springer, Berlin Heidelberg New York

Elston RC, Stewart J (1971) A general model for the genetic analysis of pedigree data. Hum Hered 21:523–542

MacCluer JW, Falk CT, Wagener DK (1985) Genetic analysis workshop III: Summary. Genet Epidemiol 2:185–198

Neugebauer M (1989) Mathematische Methoden und Algorithmen zur Analyse genetischer Polymorphismen in Stammbäumen. Inaugural-Dissertation, University of Bonn

Neugebauer M (1990) Technical Report of FAP. (in preparation)

Seuchter SA, Neugebauer M, Baur MP (1990) User manual for FAP, version 1.0

Abbreviations

AC	Adenomatosis coli	LANS	Large atypical nevus syndrome 116
AN	Atypical nevi 116		
APC	Adenomatous polyposis coli 45, 59	LINKAGE	Computer program 137, 154
BC	Breast cancer	LINKMAP	Computer program 141
CMM	Cutaneous malignant melanoma	LINKSYS	Computer program 144
		LIPED	Computer program 141, 154
CRI-MAP	Computer program 142		
dBASE	Computer program 143	LOH	Loss of heterozygosity 9, 72, 80
dGENE	Computer program 143		
DNS	Dysplastic nevus syndrome 60–61, 104, 106	MAP	Computer program 143
		MAPFUN	Computer program 143
EM	Estimation- and -maximization algorithm 150	MAPMAKER	Computer program 142
		MEN	Multiple endocrine neoplasia 5
FAMMM	Familial atypical multiple mole melanoma 114, 117	MENDEL	Computer program 143
		MLINK	Computer program 141
FAP	Familial adenomatous polyposis 11, 60	MN	Micronucleus test 117
		PAP	Computer program 141
FAP	Computer program 145	PBD	Proliferative breast disease 61
FNA	Fine-needle aspiration 61		
GPT	Glutamate-pyruvate transaminase, in breast cancer 23	PCR	Polymerase chain reaction 43
		POINTER	Computer program 19, 20–21
HBC	Hereditary breast cancer 5	RB	Retinoblastoma
		RFLP	Restriction fragment length polymorphism 9, 50, 72
HDS	Hereditary dysplastic nevus syndrome 116		
HFD	Haplotype frequency difference 90	RR	Relative risk 29, 90, 93, 106
HLA	Human leukocyte antigen 90	SCE	Sister chromatid exchange 117, 129
HNPCC	Hereditary nonpolyposis colorectal cancer 11	SEXDIF	Computer program 143
		SIMLINK	Computer program 136–137
HOMOG	Computer program 143		
ibd	Identity by descent 23, 38	SLE	Systematic Lupus erythematosum 90
ILINK	Computer program 141	SLINK	Computer program 137
ISH	In situ hybridization 67, 71, 85	WAGR	Triad in Wilms' tumor 78, 79, 82

Subject Index

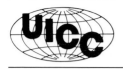 **International Union Against Cancer**

P. Hermanek, University of Erlangen-Nürnberg, Erlangen;
L. H. Sobin, Washington, D.C. (Eds.)

TNM Classification of Malignant Tumours

4th fully rev. ed. 1987. Corr. Reprint 1989. XVIII, 197 pp.
Softcover DM 22,– ISBN 3-540-17366-8

The TNM System is the most widely used classification of the extent of growth and the spread of cancer.

Specific changes in the fourth edition include:

- elimination of all differences between the AJCC (American Joint Committee on Cancer) and UICC TNM classifications of head and neck tumours and lung tumours,
- revision of the T classifications of esophageal and gastric carcinomas based on Japanese studies,
- modification of the classification of colorectal tumours to provide direct congruence with the Duke's classification and allow for a finer degree of subdivision,
- redrafting in collaboration with FIGO of the FIGO classification of gyneco-logical tumours in the format of TNM,
- addition of TNM classification for sites not previously covered in earlier UICC editions.

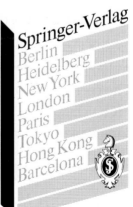

Springer-Verlag
Berlin
Heidelberg
New York
London
Paris
Tokyo
Hong Kong
Barcelona

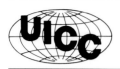 **International Union Against Cancer**

B. Spiessl, O. H. Beahrs, P. Hermanek, R. V. P. Hutter,
O. Scheibe, L. H. Sobin, G. Wagner (Eds.)

TNM Atlas

Illustrated Guide to the TNM/pTNM Classification of Malignant Tumours

Illustrations by U. Kerl

3rd ed. 1989. Corr. Reprint 1990. XIX, 343 pp. 452 figs.
Softcover DM 35,– ISBN 3-540-17721-3

The TNM classification of malignant tumours has the following objectives:
– to help the clinician in the planning of treatment,
– to determine the prognosis,
– to assist in evaluating the results of treatment,
– to facilitate the exchange of information between treatment centres,
– to contribute to the continuing investigation of human cancer.

The **TNM Atlas** is designed as an aid for the practical application of the TNM classification system.

The corrected reprint includes the latest FIGO changes in the classification for corpus uteri and vulva carcinoma.

Prices are subject to change without notice.

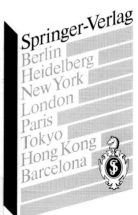